Marine Bioactive Natural Product Studies—A Southern Hemisphere Perspective

Marine Bioactive Natural Product Studies—A Southern Hemisphere Perspective

Editor

Sylvia Urban

MDPI • Basel • Beijing • Wuhan • Barcelona • Belgrade • Manchester • Tokyo • Cluj • Tianjin

Editor
Sylvia Urban
RMIT University (City Campus)
Australia

Editorial Office
MDPI
St. Alban-Anlage 66
4052 Basel, Switzerland

This is a reprint of articles from the Special Issue published online in the open access journal *Marine Drugs* (ISSN 1660-3397) (available at: https://www.mdpi.com/journal/marinedrugs/special_issues/australasian-perspective).

For citation purposes, cite each article independently as indicated on the article page online and as indicated below:

LastName, A.A.; LastName, B.B.; LastName, C.C. Article Title. *Journal Name* **Year**, *Article Number*, Page Range.

ISBN 978-3-03943-188-5 (Hbk)
ISBN 978-3-03943-189-2 (PDF)

Contents

About the Editor vii

Preface to "Marine Bioactive Natural Product Studies—A Southern Hemisphere Perspective" ix

Michael T. Davies-Coleman and Clinton G. L. Veale
Recent Advances in Drug Discovery from South African Marine Invertebrates
Reprinted from: *Mar. Drugs* **2015**, *13*, 6366–6383, doi:10.3390/md13106366 1

Kirsten Benkendorff
Natural Product Research in the Australian Marine Invertebrate *Dicathais orbita*
Reprinted from: *Mar. Drugs* **2013**, *11*, 1370–1398, doi:10.3390/md11041370 17

M. Harunur Rashid, Somayeh Mahdavi and Serdar Kuyucak
Computational Studies of Marine Toxins Targeting Ion Channels
Reprinted from: *Mar. Drugs* **2013**, *11*, 848–869, doi:10.3390/md11030848 37

Duc-Hiep Bach, Seong-Hwan Kim, Ji-Young Hong, Hyen Joo Park, Dong-Chan Oh and Sang Kook Lee
Salternamide A Suppresses Hypoxia-Induced Accumulation of HIF-1α and Induces Apoptosis in Human Colorectal Cancer Cells
Reprinted from: *Mar. Drugs* **2015**, *13*, 6962–6976, doi:10.3390/md13116962 57

Brett D. Schwartz, Mark J. Coster, Tina S. Skinner-Adams, Katherine T. Andrews, Jonathan M. White and Rohan A. Davis
Synthesis and Antiplasmodial Evaluation of Analogues Based on the Tricyclic Core of Thiaplakortones A–D
Reprinted from: *Mar. Drugs* **2015**, *13*, 55784–5795, doi:10.3390/md13095784 71

Jacquie L. Harper, Iman M. Khalil, Lisa Shaw, Marie-Lise Bourguet-Kondracki, Joëlle Dubois, Alexis Valentin, David Barker and Brent R. Copp
Structure-Activity Relationships of the Bioactive Thiazinoquinone Marine Natural Products Thiaplidiaquinones A and B
Reprinted from: *Mar. Drugs* **2015**, *13*, 5102–5110, doi:10.3390/md13085102 81

Trong D. Tran, Ngoc B. Pham, Merrick Ekins, John N. A. Hooper and Ronald J. Quinn
Isolation and Total Synthesis of Stolonines A–C, Unique Taurine Amides from the Australian Marine Tunicate *Cnemidocarpa stolonifera*
Reprinted from: *Mar. Drugs* **2015**, *13*, 4556–4575, doi:10.3390/md13074556 89

Yadollah Bahrami and Christopher M. M. Franco
Structure Elucidation of New Acetylated Saponins, Lessoniosides A, B, C, D, and E, and Non-Acetylated Saponins, Lessoniosides F and G, from the Viscera of the Sea Cucumber *Holothuria lessoni*
Reprinted from: *Mar. Drugs* **2015**, *13*, 597–617, doi:10.3390/md13010597 107

Anthony D. Wright, Jonathan L. Nielson, Dianne M. Tapiolas, Catherine H. Liptrot and Cherie A. Motti
A Great Barrier Reef *Sinularia* sp. Yields Two New Cytotoxic Diterpenes
Reprinted from: *Mar. Drugs* **2012**, *10*, 1619–1630, doi:10.3390/md10081619 125

About the Editor

Sylvia Urban is an associate professor at the School of Science, RMIT University, and a fellow of the Royal Australian Chemical Society (FRACI). She completed her PhD at The University of Melbourne and has held research appointments in the field of natural product drug discovery (with AstraZeneca and PharmaMar SA) at Griffith University and at the University of Canterbury, Christchurch, New Zealand, respectively. She was awarded an ASP Research Starter grant from the American Society of Pharmacognosy and the Gerald Blunden Award for her activities in natural product chemistry research. Her research interests include marine and terrestrial natural products chemistry; isolation and structural characterisation; NMR spectroscopy and analytical separation and profiling methodologies for natural product discovery. Sylvia leads the Marine and Terrestrial Natural Product research group at RMIT University. Sylvia is also Program Manager of the Bachelor of Science degree at RMIT University, and is a passionate chemistry educator and a leader in transforming education in STEM. In 2019, she was awarded an Australian Award for University Teaching (AAUT) Citation for Outstanding Contribution to Student Learning, and was elected as a Senior Fellow of the Higher Education Academy (SFHEA) in 2018. Sylvia has served as Deputy Chair and a committee member of the Women Researchers Network (WRN) at RMIT University, and is a committee member of the Royal Australian Chemical Society (RACI) Women in Chemistry group (WinC). Her goal is to promote better opportunities for women in science, technology, engineering and mathematics (STEM), and she has been selected for some key leadership programs that provide leadership training and support to women in the university sector. Finally, Sylvia is Reconcilation Facilitator and Ingidenous Coordinator for the School of Science at RMIT University, a role that she is passionate about, especially as it entails better understanding how we can embed indigenous knowledge into the STEM education sector.

Preface to "Marine Bioactive Natural Product Studies—A Southern Hemisphere Perspective"

The search for bioactive secondary metabolites from marine organisms has been an active area of research since the 1950s. The distinct biodiversity of the marine environment has afforded a vast array of unique secondary metabolites, many of which possess potent biological activities. This Special Issue of Marine Drugs highlights recent bioactive marine natural product studies conducted by southern hemisphere scientists on an array of marine organisms. In total, nine articles were published, covering the discovery of a range of unique marine natural products from the southern hemisphere, by implementing various strategies including synthesis, SAR studies, various isolation strategies and computational studies.

Sylvia Urban
Editor

marine drugs

MDPI

Review

Recent Advances in Drug Discovery from South African Marine Invertebrates

Michael T. Davies-Coleman [1,*] and Clinton G. L. Veale [2]

1 Department of Chemistry, University of the Western Cape, Robert Sobukwe Road, Bellville 7535, South Africa
2 Faculty of Pharmacy, Rhodes University, Grahamstown 6140, South Africa; C.Veale@ru.ac.za
* Author to whom correspondence should be addressed; mdavies-coleman@uwc.ac.za; Tel.: +27-21-959-2255.

Academic Editor: Sylvia Urban
Received: 25 July 2015; Accepted: 29 September 2015; Published: 14 October 2015

Abstract: Recent developments in marine drug discovery from three South African marine invertebrates, the tube worm *Cephalodiscus gilchristi*, the ascidian *Lissoclinum* sp. and the sponge *Topsentia pachastrelloides*, are presented. Recent reports of the bioactivity and synthesis of the anti-cancer secondary metabolites cephalostatin and mandelalides (from *C. gilchristi* and *Lissoclinum* sp., respectively) and various analogues are presented. The threat of drug-resistant pathogens, e.g., methicillin-resistant *Staphylococcus aureus* (MRSA), is assuming greater global significance, and medicinal chemistry strategies to exploit the potent MRSA PK inhibition, first revealed by two marine secondary metabolites, *cis*-3,4-dihydrohamacanthin B and bromodeoxytopsentin from *T. pachastrelloides*, are compared.

Keywords: cephalostatin; mandelalide; methicillin resistant *Staphylococcus aureus*; MRSA PK; bisindole alkaloids

1. Introduction

The plethora of intertidal and subtidal marine organisms inhabiting the *ca.* 26,000-km coastline of Africa provide a relatively untapped opportunity for the discovery of new bioactive secondary metabolites. Despite a concerted marine bio-discovery effort over the past four decades that has focused predominantly on South African marine invertebrates [1–3], only three South African marine invertebrates, *viz.* the tube worm *Cephalodiscus gilchristi*, the ascidian *Lissoclinum* sp. and the sponge *Topsentia pachastrelloides* (Figure 1), have afforded secondary metabolites whose biomedicinal potential is currently attracting international attention. Recent reports appearing in the chemical literature (June 2012–June 2015) pertaining to this cohort of secondary metabolites is overviewed. Not surprisingly, given the global problem of obtaining sufficient supplies of bioactive marine natural products from the ocean for further drug development [4], the bioactive secondary metabolites from these three South African marine invertebrates have been the subject of concerted synthetic programs geared towards producing sufficient amounts of either the natural product or potentially more bioactive analogues, for detailed biological and *in vitro* studies.

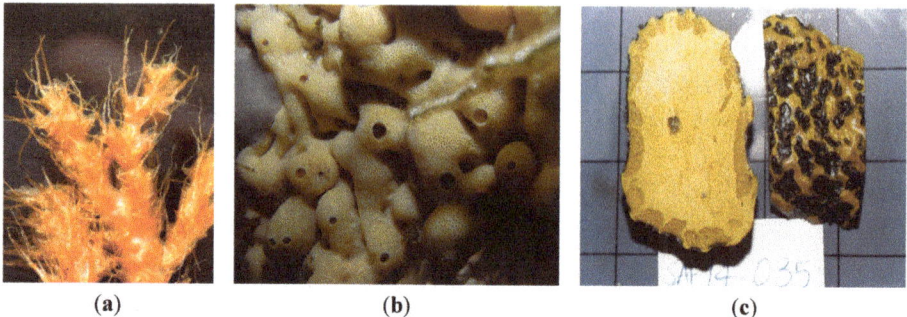

(a) **(b)** **(c)**

Figure 1. (**a**) *Cephalodiscus gilchristi* (photo: L. Lange); (**b**) *Lissoclinum* sp. (photo: S. Parker-Nance); (**c**) *Topsentia pachastrelloides* (photo: M. Davies-Coleman).

2. Tumor Growth Inhibiting Cephalostatins from the South African Marine Tube Worm *Cephalodiscus gilchristi*

The first large-scale collections of African marine invertebrates solely for the purpose of new drug discovery were coordinated by Professor G. R. Pettit of Arizona State University, USA, over three decades ago off South Africa's temperate southern coast [5]. Cephalostatin 1 (**1**, Figure 2) was isolated in low yield (*ca.* 2.3 × 10^{-7}%) from two separate and substantial SCUBA collections (166 and 450 kg (wet weight) collected in 1981 and 1990, respectively) of the hemichordate marine tube worm *Cephalodiscus gilchristi* (Figure 1a) [6]. Cephalostatin 1 has emerged as one of the most potent cell growth-inhibiting secondary metabolites ever screened by the U.S. National Cancer Institute (NCI) (ED_{50} 0.1–0.0001 pM in a P338 leukemia cell line) [6,7].

Of immediate interest to those exploring this compound's tumor growth inhibitory activities was, first, the comparative GI_{50} values (quantification of the concentration required to inhibit cellular growth by 50%) of **1** (GI_{50} 1.2 nM) with commercially available anticancer drugs, e.g., taxol (**2**, GI_{50} 29 nM), cisplatin (**3**, GI_{50} 2000 nM) and 5-fluorouracil (**4**, 24,000 nM), and, second, the 275-times higher concentration of **1** required to kill 50% of cancer cells (LC_{50} 330 nM) relative to the amount required for 50% cell growth inhibition [6]. In addition, the application of the NCI's COMPARE algorithm [8] to the GI_{50} data acquired for **1** indicated that this novel bis-steroidal pyrazine alkaloid possesses a unique mechanism of action against the proliferation of cancer cells in the NCI's *in vitro* 60 cancer cell line screen, and therefore, not surprisingly, **1** is increasingly proving to be a valuable tool for the discovery of new apoptosis signaling pathways [9]. Vollmar and co-workers' early studies into cephalostatin's apoptotic mechanism of action established that **1** promotes the release of Smac (second mitochondria-derived activator of caspase) through the dissipation of mitochondrial membrane potential [6,9,10] as part of a novel apoptosome-independent, caspase-9-mediated apoptotic pathway [6]. Furthermore, Shair and co-workers have shown that **1** also selectively binds to oxysterol binding protein (OSBP) and OSBP-related protein 4L (ORP4L) [11] and drew attention to these proteins, whose role in cancer cell survival was little known at the time. A further eighteen naturally-occurring and semi-synthetic analogues of **1** have subsequently been reported (1988–2012) in the chemical and patent literature (e.g., U.S. Patents 4873245, 5047532, 5583224 and WO 8908655). The isolation, structure elucidation, synthesis and bioactivity of this cohort of cephalostatins has been comprehensively reviewed along with the closely-related bis-steroidal pyrazine alkaloids, the ritterazines, e.g., ritterazine G, (**5**) from the Japanese ascidian (tunicate), *Ritterella tokioka* [6]. Since the publication of Iglesias-Arteaga and Morzycki's extensive review [6], the chemical structure of the twentieth member of the cephalostatin series, cephalostatin 20 (**6**), has recently been reported by Pettit *et al.* [12]. Compound **6**, the 9′-α-hydroxy analog of cephalostatin 9 (**7**), was isolated in low yield (1 × 10^{7}%) from the combined bioactive (cytotoxic to P338 murine lymphocyte cells) fractions from the original extract of *C. gilchristi* [5] nearly a quarter of a century ago. Interestingly, the cell growth inhibitory activities of **6** and **7** against six human tumor cell lines was 100–1000-times less active than **1** in the same tumor cell panel, thus underlining the importance of an intact spirostanol structure in the southern unit of cephalostatins to the growth inhibition activities of these compounds [12].

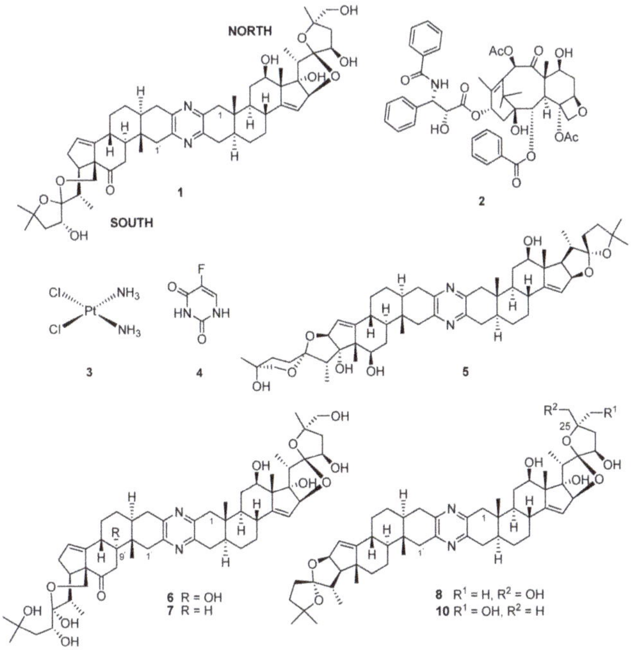

Figure 2. Chemical structures of compounds **1–8** and **10**.

Significant effort [6,13,14] has been directed towards the total enantioselective syntheses of **1** over the last two decades. Following on from their first 65-step convergent total synthesis of **1** and potently active cephalostatin/ritterazine hybrids [15], Fuchs and co-workers have recently reported the first convergent total synthesis of 25-*epi* ritterostatin G_N1_N **8** [16] from commercially available dihydroxyhecogenin acetate (**9**, Figure 3). Fuchs and co-workers identified the key step in their synthesis as a chiral ligand ($(DHQ)_2$PHAL)-mediated dihydroxylation reaction, which introduced the 25-*epi* functionality into the north segment (analogous to the north unit of cephalostatin) [16]. Compound **8**, structurally incorporating the north units of both **1** and **5**, exhibited a mean GI_{50} (0.48 nM) in a panel of eight cancer cell lines and was 30-fold more active than ritterostatin (**10**), also screened in the same cell line panel [16].

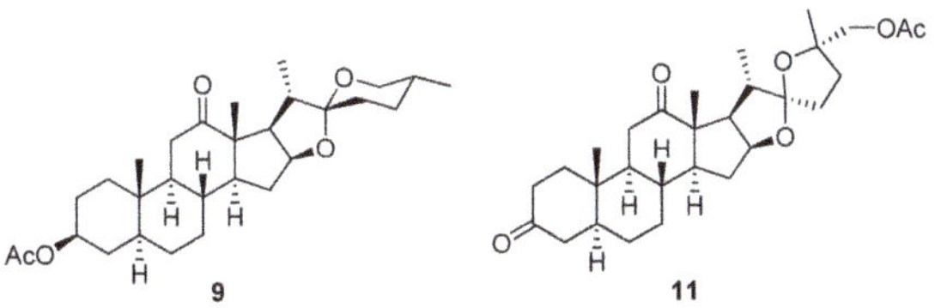

Figure 3. Chemical structures of synthetic intermediates **9** and **11**.

The daunting synthetic challenges of cephalostatin molecular architecture continue to inspire the synthesis of simpler analogs with similar bioactivities to **1** [6]. The latest target in this series, [5.5]-spiroketal (**11**, Figure 3), which shares the steroidal scaffold of the northern hemisphere of **1** with an intact 1,6-dioxaspiro[5.5]nonane side chain, but with a diminished oxygenation pattern, was synthesized by Pettit *et al.* in seven steps from **9** in an overall 4.6% yield [17]. Although **11** and several synthetic precursors of this compound were not cytotoxic to P388 leukemia cells, Pettit *et al.* suggested that **9** was potentially useful as a synthetically-accessible starting point for further synthetic modification into both symmetrical and asymmetrical trisdecacyclic bis-steroidal pyrazine congeners of **1** [17] through well-established pyrazine ring construction protocols [16].

3. Synthesis and Revision of the Absolute Configuration of the Cytotoxic Mandelalides from the South African Marine Ascidian, *Lissoclinum* sp.

The encrusting colonial didemnid ascidian *Lissoclinum* sp. (Figure 1b) collected by SCUBA from Algoa Bay, on the southeast coast of South Africa, afforded sub-milligram (0.5–0.8 mg) quantities of the glycosylated, polyketide macrolides, the mandelalides A–D (**12a**, **13–15**, Figure 4). Mandelalides A and B exhibited potent low nanomolar cytotoxicity (IC_{50} 12 and 44 nM, respectively) against NCI-H460 lung cancer cells [18]. The relative configuration of the macrolide rings in **12a**, **13–15** was established through integration of ROESY data with homonuclear ($^3J_{HH}$) and heteronuclear ($^{2,3}J_{CH}$) coupling constants, while the absolute configurations of **12a** and **13** were extrapolated from the hydrolysis and subsequent chiral GC-MS analysis of the respective monosaccharide residues (2-*O*-methyl-6-dehydro-α-L-rhamnose and 2-*O*-methyl-6-dehydro-α-L-talose). The paucity of **12a**, **13–15** isolated from the MeOH-CH_2Cl_2 extract of *Lissoclinum* sp. (*i.e.*, 0.8 mg of **12a**) and difficulties encountered in the further supply of these compounds from their natural source implied that the synthesis of **12a** (the most active compound in the mandelalide series) would provide sufficient quantities of **12a** to explore the mechanism of *in vitro* cytotoxicity exhibited by this compound. As described below, the synthesis of **12a** and the diastereomer **16** by Willwacher *et al.* and Xu, Ye and co-workers revealed errors in the original assignment of the absolute configuration at positions C17, C18 C20, C21 and C23 and resulted in the correction of the chemical structure of mandelalide A (**12a**) to **16** [19,20].

In 2014, two years after the isolation of the mandelalides was first reported [18], Willwacher and Fürstner reported the first total synthesis of **12a** in a 4.5% overall yield [21]. They also noted the structural similarities between **12a** and madeirolide A (**17**, Figure 4), an equally scarce metabolite previously isolated from a marine sponge, *Leiodermatium* sp. [22,23], and ascribed the absence of anti-proliferative activity against pancreatic cancer cells reported for **17** to the structural differences between these two compounds. Anticipating in their proposed synthesis of **12a** that final closure of the macrolide ring, concomitant with insertion of the Δ^{14} *Z*-olefin, could be achieved with ring closing alkyne metathesis (RCAM), Willwacher and Fürstner successfully synthesized the two main building blocks (**18**) and (**19**) emerging from their retrosynthetic analysis of **12a**. Cobalt-catalyzed carbonylative epoxide opening and iridium-catalyzed two-directional Krische allylation were identified as key synthetic steps required for the synthesis of **18** and **19**, respectively, while the RCAM protocol would not have been possible without the use of a highly-selective molybdenum alkylidene complex catalyst; the first time that this catalyst has been successfully incorporated into a natural product total synthesis [21]. Finally, regioselective trimethylsilyl trifluoromethanesulfonate (TESOTf)-catalyzed rhamnosylation of the mandelalide aglycone proceeded smoothly to afford mandelalide A with the chemical structure **12a**, originally proposed by McPhail and co-workers [18].

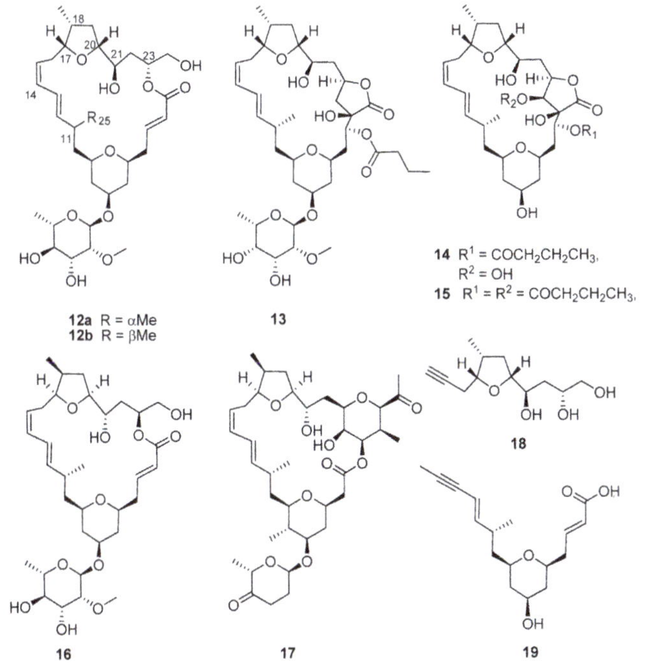

Figure 4. Chemical structures of compounds **12a–19**.

Comparing the spectroscopic data acquired for their synthetic product with those of naturally-occurring mandelalide A (**16**), Willwacher and Fürstner noted significant chemical shift and coupling constant differences between the NMR datasets of synthetic **12a** and the natural product (Tables 1 and 2). Initially, given the relative magnitude of the observed differences, their attention was focused on differences in the ^{13}C chemical shift assigned to the C11 methine and the C25 methyl carbon atoms (Table 1) and discrepancies in the $^{3}J_{11,12}$ coupling constants (Table 2; $J_{11,12}$ = 9.7 and 7.6 Hz, respectively, for naturally-occurring mandelalide A and **12a**, respectively) associated with the C11 stereogenic center. However, synthesis of the 11-*epi*-diastereomer of **12a** (**12b**) did not provide clarity on the source of spectroscopic differences between the synthetic and natural products, and Willwacher and Fürstner were at a loss to explain where the anomalies resided in the proposed structure of **12a** [21]. Reddy *et al.* [24] also tackled the synthesis of the aglycone of **12a**, reflected in the original structure proposed by McPhail and co-workers [18]. Their 32-step synthesis afforded the putative mandelalide A aglycone in a 6.3% overall yield, and the spectroscopic data acquired for the synthetic product was consistent with the analogous data for the aglycone of **12a** synthesized by Willwacher and Fürstner.

Table 1. Comparative ^{13}C NMR data ($CDCl_3$, 175 † and 150 ‡ MHz) reported by McPhail and co-workers [18] for naturally-occurring **16**; by Willwacher *et al.* [20,21] for synthetic **12a**, **12b** and **16**; and by Xu, Ye and co-workers [19] for synthetic **12a** and **16**.

Carbon	Naturally-Occurring 16 [18] †	Synthetic 12a [21] ‡	Synthetic 12b [21] ‡	Synthetic 12a [19] ‡	Synthetic 16 [19] ‡	Synthetic 16 [20] ‡
1	167.4	167.3	166.8	167.1	167.4	167.4
2	123.1	123.1	123.6	122.9	123.0	123.1
3	147.1	146.3	146.1	146.2	147.2	147.1
4	38.8	38.5	39.5	38.2	38.8	38.8
5	73.9	73.4	73.9	73.2	73.9	73.9
6	37.6	36.7	38.2	36.4	37.6	37.6
7	73.1	72.8	72.7	72.6	73.1	73.1
8	39.7	39.3	39.2	39.0	39.7	39.7
9	72.5	73.1	73.2	72.9	72.5	72.5
10	43.1	42.9	43.5	42.6	43.1	43.1
11	34.2	32.8	34.1	32.6	34.2	34.2
12	141.5	140.9	141.3	140.6	141.6	141.5
13	123.9	123.8	124.9	123.6	123.9	123.9
14	131.3	130.5	130.6	130.3	131.3	131.3
15	126.9	126.5	126.2	126.3	127.0	126.9
16	31.1	31.2	31.0	31.0	31.1	31.1
17	81.0	81.3	81.8	81.1	81.0	81.0
18	37.3	37.1	36.9	36.9	37.4	37.4
19	36.8	36.0	36.4	35.8	36.8	36.8
20	83.2	82.7	82.1	82.5	83.2	83.2
21	73.0	73.4	73.3	72.3	73.0	73.1
22	34.1	34.1	34.7	33.9	34.1	34.1
23	72.3	72.5	74.0	72.3	72.3	72.3
24	66.1	65.7	65.7	65.6	66.1	66.1
25	18.3	20.1	22.0	19.9	18.3	18.3
26	14.5	14.7	14.9	14.6	14.6	14.5
1′	94.2	94.0	94.1	93.7	94.2	94.2
2′	80.8	80.9	80.9	80.6	80.8	80.8
3′	71.7	71.7	71.6	71.4	71.7	71.7
4′	74.3	74.2	74.2	74.0	74.3	74.3
5′	68.1	68.2	68.2	67.9	68.1	68.1
6′	17.7	17.7	17.7	17.5	17.7	17.7
7′	59.1	59.2	59.1	59.0	59.2	59.1

Table 2. Comparative ^{1}H NMR data ($CDCl_3$, 700 † and 600 ‡ MHz) reported by McPhail and co-workers [18] for naturally-occurring **16** and by Willwacher *et al.* [20,21] for synthetic **12a** and **16**.

	Naturally-Occurring 16 [18] †			**Synthetic 12a [21] ‡**			**Synthetic 16 [20] ‡**		
No.	δ (ppm)	mult.	*J* (Hz)	δ (ppm)	mult.	*J* (Hz)	δ (ppm)	mult.	*J* (Hz)
1									
2	6.01	dd	15.5, 1.2	5.92	dt	15.6, 1.5	6.01	dt	15.5, 0.8
3	6.97	ddd	15.2, 10.4, 4.6	7.02	ddd	15.5, 8.6, 5.5	6.96	ddd	15.3, 10.4, 4.9
4a	2.36	m		2.34	dddd	15.2, 6.5, 5.6, 1.8	2.36	m	
4b	2.39	ddd	14.1, 10.6, 10.6	2.46	dddd	15.2, 8.6, 3.7, 1.2	2.39	ddd	13.9, 10.8, 10.7
5	3.36	dddd	11.4, 11.4, 2.3, 2.3	3.42	m		3.37	m	
6a	1.20	m		1.26	m		1.20	m	
6b	2.02	dddd	12.6, 4.4, 2.3, 1.6	1.94	ddt	12.0, 4.6, 1.9	2.02	dddd	12.1, 5.6, 2.3, 1.6
7	3.82	dddd	11.1, 10.5, 4.4, 4.4	3.77	m		3.82	dddd	11.3, 10.6, 4.8, 4.5
8a	1.22	m		1.22	m		1.22	m	
8b	1.87	m		1.84	dddd	12.5, 4.2, 1.9, 1.9	1.87	dddt	13.2, 7.8, 5.3, 1.9
9	3.32	dddd	11.2, 11.2, 2.2, 2.2	3.33	m		3.31	tt	10.7, 2.1
10a	1.21	ddd	15.2, 9.6, 2.2	1.27	m		1.21	m	
10b	1.51	ddd	15.2, 11.2, 3.7	1.69	ddd	14.1, 9.1, 5.1	1.52	ddd	14.1, 11.1, 3.3
11	2.37	dqd	9.6, 6.5, 3.7	2.44	m		2.37	m	
12	5.45	dd	14.8, 9.7	5.61	dd	15.2, 7.6	5.44	dd	14.9, 9.9
13	6.28	dd	14.8, 9.7	6.22	ddt	15.2, 10.8, 1.0	6.27	dd	14.8, 11.1
14	6.05	dd	10.9, 10.9	6.01	tt	10.8, 1.8	6.05	dd	10.9, 10.9
15	5.28	ddd	10.8, 10.8, 5.6	5.27	ddd	10.8, 8.3, 7.5	5.28	dt	10.8, 5.6
16a	1.88	m		2.14	dddd	14.8, 6.8, 5.1, 1.9	1.88	m	
16b	2.28	ddd	13.1, 11.4, 11.4	2.29	dtd	14.8, 8.5, 1.6	2.25	m	
17	3.98	ddd	11.1, 8.1, 1.8	4.03	ddd	8.6, 7.2, 4.9	3.98	ddd	10.9, 8.5, 1.7
18	2.52	dddq	12.0, 7.0, 7.0	2.43	m		2.52	dddq	12.3, 7.0, 7.0, 6.9
19a	1.17	ddd	11.9, 11.9, 10.3	1.28	m		1.17	ddd	12.2, 12.1, 10.2
19b	2.01	ddd	12.2, 7.0, 5.6	2.04	dt	12.3, 6.7	2.01	ddd	11.8, 7.1, 6.0
20	3.63	m		3.71	ddd	8.4, 8.2, 6.7	3.63	m	
21	3.42	ddd	11.1, 8.8, 1.8	3.45	m		3.42	ddd	11.2, 8.9, 1.8
22a	1.46	ddd	14.1, 11.1, 1.9	1.54	ddd	14.4, 10.5, 2.5	1.46	ddd	14.2, 11.3, 1.9
22b	1.76	ddd	13.9, 11.7, 1.8	1.77	ddd	14.4, 10.8, 2.0	1.76	ddt	12.8, 12.6, 1.5
23	5.23	dddd	11.7, 4.9, 2.9, 1.9	5.24	m		5.23	dddd	11.6, 5.1, 3.1, 2.0
24a	3.61	m		3.65	m		3.61	m	
24b	3.81	dd	12.1, 2.9	3.78	dd	12.1, 3.3	3.79	m	
25	0.85	d	6.6	1.00	d	6.7	0.85	d	6.6
26	1.03	d	6.9	0.98	d	7.0	1.02	d	7.0
1′	5.02	d	1.1	5.02	d	1.5	5.02	d	1.1
2′	3.40	dd	3.8, 1.4	3.40	dd	3.8, 1.5	3.40	dd	3.4, 1.5
3′	3.68	m		3.69	m		3.68	td	9.8, 3.7
4′	3.34	dd	9.4, 9.4	3.34	t	9.4	3.34	dd	10.5, 9.3
5′	3.62	m		3.63	dd	9.4, 6.1	3.62	dd	9.9, 5.9
6′	1.27	d	6.3	1.28	d	6.3	1.26	d	6.3
7′	3.45	s		3.46	s		3.45	s	
OH-1′				2.45–2.33			2.69	br s	
OH-2′				2.56–2.33			2.31	br s	
OH-3′	2.24	s		2.44–2.34			2.35	m	
OH-4′	1.54	s		2.78–2.64	br s		2.53	br s	

A second synthesis of **12a** by Xu, Ye and co-workers [19] was published in Angewandte Chemie International Edition shortly after Willwacher and Fürstner's synthetic communication appeared in the same volume of the journal. Approaching the synthesis of the 24-membered macrocycle via a different route to that used by Willwacher and Fürstner; Xu, Ye and co-workers initially constructed the two sub-units (**20** and **21**, Figure 5) with Prins cyclization, providing diastereoselective access to the tetrahydropyran moiety in **20** and a Rychnovsky–Bartlett cyclization generating the tetrahydrofuran ring in **21**. As anticipated from the retrosynthetic analysis that guided this synthetic approach, both subunits were successfully assembled into the aglycone via Suzuki coupling and Horner–Wadsworth–Emmons macrocyclization. The synthesis of **12a** was concluded with the addition of a protected rhamnose moiety to the mandelalide aglycone via a Kahne glycosylation reaction followed by a single-step collective removal of the silyl protecting groups. Xu, Ye and co-workers also identified the incompatibility of the NMR datasets acquired for their synthetic product and naturally-occurring mandelalide A, including the significant chemical shift differences associated with the C11 and C25 carbon atoms (Tables 1 and 2). However, from direct comparison of the opposite configurations of the stereogenic centers in the northern hemisphere of **12a** and **17**, they correctly postulated that, assuming **12a** and **17** share a common biogenesis, the differences in absolute configuration would probably be confined to this part of the molecule and not C11, to which an *S* configuration was assigned in both **12a** and **17**. The convergent synthetic approach to **12a** by Xu, Ye and co-workers enabled them to synthesize the diastereomer, **16**, with opposite configurations at positions C17, C18 C20, C21 and C23 to those initially reported for **12a** [18] and consistent with the configurations assigned to the analogous chiral centers in **17** [19]. Willwacher *et al.* also recently reported a further synthesis of **16** [20] and confidently postulated revised structures for mandelalide B–D (**22–24**, Figure 5). Comparison of the NMR data of naturally-occurring mandelalide A with those of **16** (Tables 1 and 2) confirmed that these two compounds were identical and that any uncertainties around the correct structure of mandelalide A had been successfully resolved.

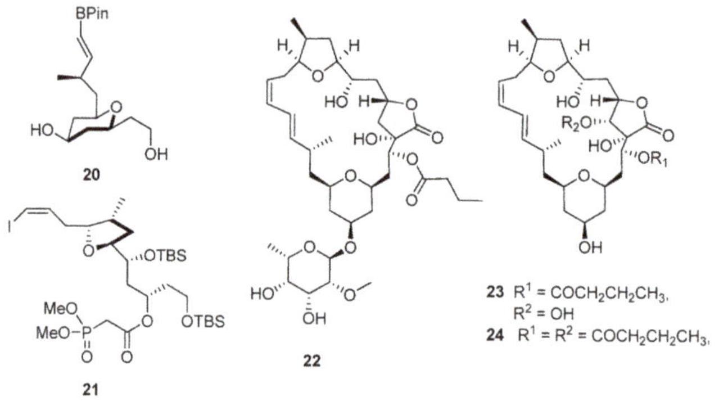

Figure 5. Chemical structures of compounds **20–25**.

Although the chemical structure of mandelalide A has now been unequivocally established as **16**, the inconsistency in the cytotoxicity data reported for this compound remains unresolved. McPhail and co-workers reported that the naturally-occurring mandelalides A and B possessed potent cytotoxicity against human NCI-H460 lung cancer cells (IC_{50} 12 and 44 nM, respectively) and Neuro-2A neuroblastoma cells (IC_{50} 29 and 84 nM, respectively) [18]. These results are at variance with the reported lack of cytotoxicity exhibited by synthetic **16** when screened against a panel of ten cancer cell lines of different histological origin by Xu, Ye and co-workers [19] (Table 3). Willwacher *et al.* also noted the negligible cytotoxicity of **16** against cancer cell lines with the exception of a single human breast carcinoma cell line [20] (Table 3).

Table 3. Comparative IC_{50} data (μM) reported by McPhail and co-workers [18] for naturally-occurring **16** and by Xu, Ye and co-workers [19] and Willwacher *et al.* [20] for synthetic **16**.

Cell Line	Histological Origin	Naturally-Occurring 16 [18]	Synthetic 16 [19]	Synthetic 16 [20]
Neuro-2A	Neuro	0.044		
NCI-H460	Lung	0.012		
H1299	Lung		25.5	
PC-3	Prostate		108.7	
PLC/PRF/5	Liver		140.6	
MHCC97L	Liver		>500	
HeLa	Cervix		249.0	
SH-SY5Y	Brain		>500	
HCT 116	Colon		>500	
HT-29	Colon		>500	>1000
MCF7	Breast		271.5	
MDA-MB-361-DYT2	Breast			0.041
N87	Stomach			0.206

4. Bisindole Alkaloid Inhibitors of Methicillin-Resistant *Staphylococcus aureus* Pyruvate Kinase from the South African Marine Sponge *Topsentia* sp.

Methicillin-resistant *Staphylococcus aureus* (MRSA), euphemistically also referred to as the "super bug", was initially encountered in public healthcare facilities and remains a significant cause of mortality in these facilities. MRSA is no longer confined to healthcare facilities and has been increasingly reported from the general population and domestic livestock worldwide [25–27]. Annually, MRSA accounts for *ca.* 94,000 infections and 18,000 deaths in the USA and 150,000 infections in the EU [27]. There are no available MRSA mortality data from Southern Africa. However, a 2015 study conducted in three South African academic hospitals reported a MRSA prevalence rate (MRSA infections as a % of all recorded *S. aureus* infections) of 36%, which is comparable to Israel (33.5%) Ireland (38.1%) and the U.K. (35.5%) [28]. The escalating infection and mortality rates associated with the ongoing spread of drug-resistant pathogenic bacteria, e.g., MRSA, are further exacerbated by the dearth of new antibiotics entering the clinic [29].

Paradoxically, the targeting of bacteria-specific proteins in new antibacterial drug development programs is problematic given the concomitant selective pressure that drugs, emerging from this classic drug discovery approach, exert on the pathogens, leading to the proliferation of drug-resistant bacterial strains [30]. Protein target-based antibiotic drug discovery is, however, not redundant. Contemporary genomic and proteomic studies of MRSA [31,32] have increased our understanding of the complex protein-protein interaction networks (interactomes) in this organism. The detailed mapping of interactomes has led to the identification of highly-connected hub proteins, which, given their centrality within the interactomes, are essential for mediating key cellular processes and sustaining MRSA viability [30,31]. Out of necessity, hub proteins are evolutionarily-conserved proteins, given the deleterious effect that mutations of hub proteins would have on the complex interactomes in which they play a key role [30]. Therefore, targeting hub proteins within the MRSA interactomes will minimize the potential for the emergence of drug resistance in MRSA and is a novel strategy for developing much needed new chemotherapeutic interventions against this drug-resistant pathogen [31]. Amongst the suite of hub proteins in a 608-protein interactome network (comprising 23% of the proteome in a hospital-acquired strain of MRSA), Zoraghi *et al.* identified pyruvate kinase (PK) as a suitable target for possible antibiotic drug discovery [30]. Catalyzing the rate-limiting irreversible conversion of phosphoenolpyruvate into pyruvate during glycolysis, pyruvate kinases are, not surprisingly, ubiquitous in both prokaryotes and eukaryotes. Fortuitously, the MRSA PK homotetramer (Figure 6a) has several possible lipophilic binding pockets that are absent in human PK orthologs, allowing potential selective inhibition of this enzyme target [33]. Initially, two parallel strategies were used to generate lead compounds to exploit the inhibition of this key enzyme. The first strategy involved the random screening of >900 marine invertebrate extracts, including those from South African marine invertebrates, for selective MRSA PK inhibition. The second rational drug design strategy coupled knowledge of the detailed structure of the MRSA PK enzyme binding site with contemporary computer-aided drug design techniques to generate new synthetic MRSA PK inhibitors. Both strategies are reviewed in more detail below.

The random screening of 968 marine invertebrate extracts, collected from seven different benthic marine environments around the world, [34], afforded only one extract that was active in the MRSA PK inhibition assay. The methanolic extract of the South African sponge, *Topsentia pachastrelloides* (Figure 1c), showed significant activity in the MRSA PK inhibition assay, and subsequent bioassay-guided fractionation of this extract yielded a cohort of four bisindole alkaloids of which, the two known metabolites *cis*-3,4-dihydrohamacanthin B (**25**, Figure 7) and bromodeoxytopsentin (**26**) proved to be the most active compounds (IC_{50} 16 and 60 nM, respectively). These two compounds also exhibited between 166- and 600-fold selectivity for MRSA PK when compared to similar inhibition data acquired from screening **25** and **26** against four human PK orthologs. X-ray crystallographic analysis of the co-crystallized *cis*-3,4-dihydrohamacanthin B-MRSA PK complex revealed that **25** was neither bound to the recognized activation nor allosteric effector binding sites on this enzyme, but was instead unexpectedly bound to two identical lipophilic binding sites on the small interface of the MRSA PK homotetramer [34].

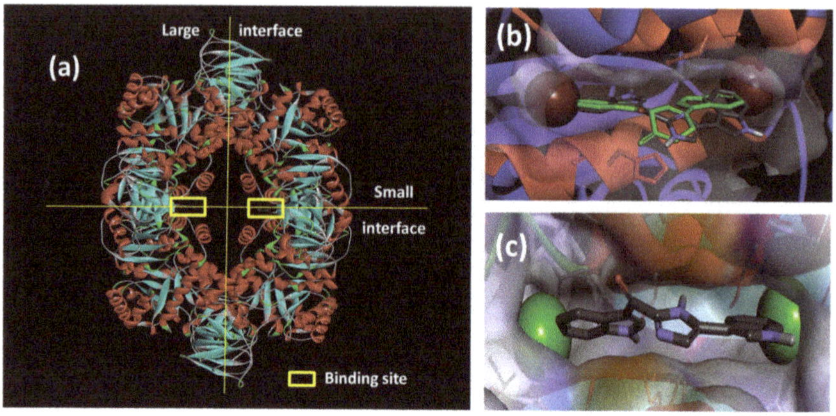

Figure 6. (**a**) X-ray structure of MRSA PK (PDB Accession Number 3T07) with the large and small interfaces and the *cis*-3,4-dihydrohamacanthin B binding sites indicated; (**b**) X-ray co-crystal generated diagram of **25** (green) in the *cis*-3,4-dihydrohamacanthin B binding site of MRSA PK with **26** (grey) overlaid in its highest scoring docked conformation with its bromines displayed as CPK models; (**c**) highest scoring docked conformation of the synthetic compound **33**, with its chlorines displayed as CPK models, in the MRSA PK *cis*-3,4-dihydrohamacanthin B binding site.

The small interface in MRSA PK is postulated to be crucial for establishing the rigidity of MRSA PK necessary for catalytic activity, and the binding of either **25** or **26** to this region of the protein is therefore thought to induce flexibility and, subsequently, to reduce enzyme activity [33]. The symmetrical *cis*-3,4-dihydrohamacanthin B binding sites are characterized by two lipophilic pockets with an appropriate spatial arrangement to readily accommodate the bromine substituents of **25** and **26** (Figure 6b). In addition, the histidine residues (HIS365) on the neighboring parallel MRSA PK α-helices rearrange to anchor the indole rings through π-interactions [34,35]. Interestingly, sequence alignment between MRSA and human PK isoforms indicated that access to the analogous binding sites in human PK orthologs is hindered by a group of amino acids that effectively shield these sites from potential ligands [33]. This structural difference around the entrance to the binding sites is consequently thought to account for the greater selectivity of **25** and **26**, and related synthetic inhibitors *vide infra*, for MRSA PK over human PK orthologs [33,35].

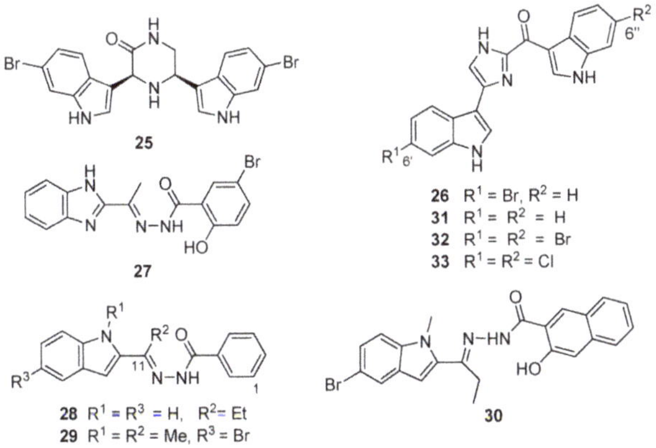

Figure 7. Chemical structures of compounds **25**–**33**.

From the preliminary screening of an *in silico* library, coupled with functional enzyme assays, Zoraghi *et al.* identified the benzimidazole compound IS-130 (**27**, Figure 7) as a potent MRSA PK inhibitor (IC_{50} 91 nM) with good specificity (>1000-fold) for MRSA PK over human isoforms, but with poor *in vivo* antibacterial activity at the cellular level against a methicillin-susceptible strain of *S. aureus* (MSSA) (minimum inhibitory concentration (MIC) >187 μg/mL) [30]. Nevertheless, the structural motif of **27** provided the starting point for a medicinal chemistry program aimed at improving selectivity, potency and antibacterial activity of potential MRSA PK inhibitors. Compound AM-168 (**28**) exhibited only slightly reduced potency (IC_{50} 126 nM) and substantially increased antibacterial activity (MIC 9.7 μg/mL), which was attributed by Zoraghi *et al.* to increased cell membrane penetration due to the increased lipophilicity imparted by the C11 ethyl substituent to this compound [30]. Accordingly, additional alkyl substitution, e.g., NSK5-15 (**29**), further enhanced antibacterial activity against several strains of MSSA and MRSA (MIC 1.4–5.8 μg/mL) with a further decrease in MRSA PK inhibitory potency (185 nM). Kumar *et al.* [33] extended Zoraghi *et al.*'s preliminary study and prepared a series of >70 compounds in which systematic structural changes were made to the heteroaromatic ring, the phenolic moiety and the central linker unit of the hit compound **27**. This series of compounds was screened against MRSA PK and methicillin-susceptible *S. aureus*, with Kumar *et al.* reporting varying levels of potency (IC_{50} 15–380 nM) and antibacterial activity (MIC 1–>194 μg/mL), respectively. Interestingly, co-crystallization of **27** and **28** with MRSA PK followed by X-ray analysis revealed that these compounds were also bound to the *cis*-3,4-dihydrohamacanthin B binding sites of the MRSA PK enzyme (Figure 6a) [33]. Unfortunately, Kumar *et al.*'s synthetic program did not shed any light on the structure activity relationships that might conclusively link potency (IC_{50}) with antibacterial activity (MIC). Ultimately, *N*-methylindole (**30**) provided the best combination of *in vitro* MRSA PK inhibition (IC_{50} 79 nM) and antibacterial activity (MIC 1 μg/mL), possibly warranting further exploitation of **30** and analogous compounds as potential antibiotics effective against MRSA [33].

Veale *et al.* [35] used the chemical structure of the naturally-occurring hit compound **26** identified in the South African sponge extract as a starting point for an extensive ligand-receptor docking study of various analogs of **26** with the *cis*-3,4-dihydrohamacanthin B binding site. Postulating that a dihalogenated analog of **26** would better exploit the opportunities offered by the symmetrical *cis*-3,4-dihydrohamacanthin B binding site, in particular the two terminal lipophilic binding pockets, Veale *et al.* prepared the 6′, 6″dihalogenated (F, Cl, Br and I, Figure 7) analogues of **26** and the debrominated compound, deoxytopsentin (**31**), for a comparative MRSA PK inhibition study. The target halogenated synthetic compounds were readily accessed in reasonable overall yield (10%–32% over five steps) via the dehydrative cyclocondensation of the respective *N*-Boc-protected 6-halo-indolyl-3-glyoxals with ammonium acetate in ethanol, followed by thermolytic cleavage of the *N*-Boc groups. As expected, the MRSA inhibition activity of the non-halogenated compound **31** (IC_{50} 240 nM) was less active than the naturally-occurring monobrominated compound **26** (IC_{50} 60 nM), while both the dibrominated and dichlorinated (Figure 6c) analogs (**32** and **33**) were an order of magnitude more potent (IC_{50} 2 and 1.5 nM, respectively) than **26** coupled to improved selectivity for MRSA PK over the four human orthologs assayed [35].

Veale *et al.* further evaluated the importance of the imidazole ring to MRSA PK inhibition in dihalogenated bisindole alkaloids by preparing a similar series of dihalogenated bisindoles in which the imidazole ring was replaced by a thiazole moiety, e.g., **34** [36] (Figure 8). Coupling of α-oxo-1*H*-indole-3-thioacetamide (**35**) with the α-bromoketone (**36**) in a regiospecific Hantzsch thiazole ring formation reaction afforded the targeted halogenated bisindole thiazoles. The μM activity of the synthetic bisindole thiazoles (e.g., IC_{50} 5 μM for **35**) indicated that bioisosteric replacement of the imidazole ring with a thiazole had a negative impact on MRSA PK potency [36]. The antibacterial activity of both the synthetic bisindole imidazoles and bisindole thiazoles was not recorded.

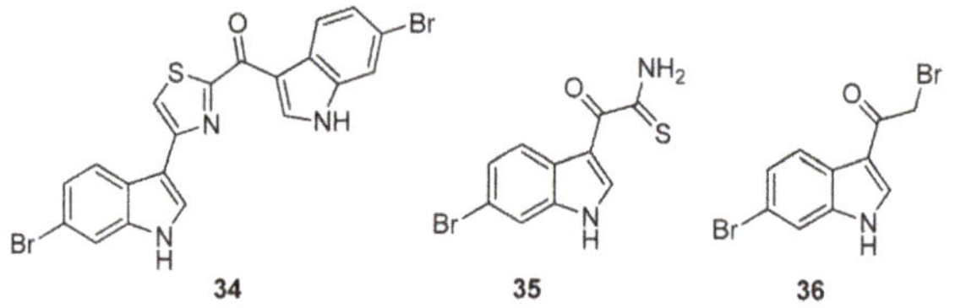

Figure 8. Chemical structures of compounds **34–36**.

Furthermore, acknowledging the significance of a bisindole motif to increased inhibition of MRSA PK, Sperry and co-workers have recently described the selective MRSA PK inhibition of a cohort of eleven, variously-substituted, synthetic 1,2-bis(3-indolyly)ethane compounds, e.g., **37** [37] (Figure 9). Compound **37**, accessed via palladium catalyzed heteroannulation of the aldehyde (**38**) and 1-iodo-2-amino-4-nitrobenzene (**39**) [38], was the most potent of the series (IC_{50} 0.9 μM) and exhibited a 20–106-fold selectivity for MRSA PK over four human PK isoforms. Replacing the C6 nitro substituent with chloro, nitrile, methoxy and methyl functionalities had a deleterious effect on MRSA PK inhibition, with the nitrile and methoxy analogs inactive and the chloro and methyl analogs two orders of magnitude less active (IC_{50} 272 and 294 μM, respectively) [37].

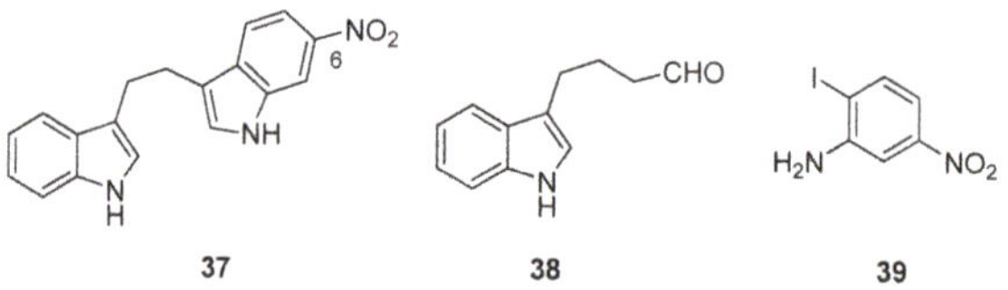

Figure 9. Chemical structures of compounds **37–39**.

Similarly, Kumar *et al.* [39] changed direction from their earlier medicinal chemistry program based on the putative MRSA PK inhibitor, **27**, to focus on potential bisindole inhibitors of MRSA PK in line with the chemical structures of the potent naturally-occurring bisindole MRSA PK inhibitors, **25** and **26**. Central to their strategy was varying the linker units between the indole rings in order to uncover the relationship between activity and indole orientation relative to the linker unit in addition to providing further insight into size constraints within the MRSA PK binding site. Their initial cohort of directly-linked 2,2′-biindoles (**40–42**, Figure 10) was synthesized through a Suzuki–Miyaura coupling of boronic acid precursor **43** and iodinated indole **44**. This cohort of compounds were generally found to potently inhibit MRSA PK at concentrations as low as 1 nM. Initial inhibitory data obtained by Kumar *et al.* supported previous observations made between deoxytopsentin analogues **26** and

32 that 6-6′ dibrominated bisindoles, such as 40 (IC_{50} 7 nM), display superior MRSA PK inhibition than a corresponding monobrominated analogue, e.g., **41** (IC_{50} 21 nM). However, the opposite trend was observed with regard to MIC values (16 and 2 μg/mL, respectively) against MSSA strains [39]. Interestingly, the 6,5′ dibrominated analogue (**42**) also displayed potent MRSA PK inhibition (IC_{50} 2.2 nM) coupled to a significantly improved MIC against *S. aureus* (0.3 μg/mL). The structure activity relationship of the linker group between indoles was further explored through insertion of acetylene, ethylene and ethyl moieties between the two substituted indole rings (**45–48**, Figure 10) using standard synthetic protocols. Similar MPSA PK inhibitory activity was observed between this group and the 2,2′-biindoles. However, MIC activity against *S. aureus* was generally lost, with the single exception of the 6,5′ dibrominated analogue **46**. An additional set of aryl linked bisindole analogues (**49–52**) were prepared with a view toward exploiting possible interactions with the aromatic histidine residues present in the binding site. The dibrominated compound (**49**) was found to be comparatively less active than compound **40**, while activity was restored with the mono-brominated compound (**50**), leading the authors to suggest that Compound **50** defines the maximum permissible length within the MRSA PK binding site. Interestingly, analogues of **50** featuring substitutions on the aryl ring (**51, 52**) were found to be the most active in the series against MRSA PK (IC_{50} *ca.* 2 nM) while the nitro-containing compound **52** showed encouraging activity against *S. aureus* (MIC 2.0 μg/mL). While no conclusive rationale for the differences between MRSA PK inhibitory activity and MIC values was postulated, Kumar *et al.* determined, through co-administration of their synthetic compounds with the calcium channel blocker verapamil (**53**), that several bisindoles were actively removed from the cells via cellular efflux mechanisms, possibly accounting for the contrasting antibacterial activities observed in their study [39].

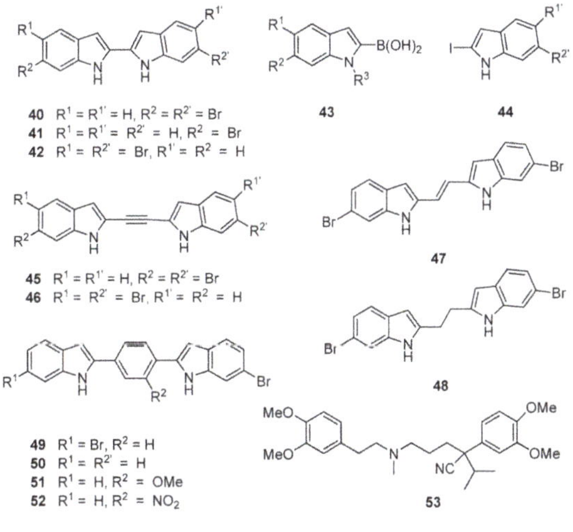

Figure 10. Chemical structures of compounds **40–53**.

5. Conclusions

Interest from Pettit and others in the anti-cancer potential of **1** has remained undiminished for nearly three decades and is likely to continue for the foreseeable future. Realization of the true potential and possible further drug development of the cephalostatins has been hampered by access to commercially-viable synthesis of sufficient quantities of either **1** or similarly-bioactive congeners. Although accessible by laboratory synthesis, potential future drug development interest in **16** will only resume if conflicting cancer cell cytotoxicity data reported for naturally-occurring and synthetic **16** can be explained. The negative impact of drug-resistant pathogens, e.g., MRSA on human health is steadily increasing, and the need for new antibiotics against these pathogens is continually emphasized. Although the *cis*-3,4-dihydrohamacanthin B binding site of MRSA PK has been identified as a potential selective anti-biotic drug target, resolving the conundrum between potent MRSA PK inhibition and poor *in vivo* MRSA antibacterial activity will define the future of this approach to MRSA antibiotic drug discovery.

Acknowledgments: The authors acknowledge with gratitude the ongoing support for South African marine bio-discovery by the South African National Research Foundation, Department of Environmental Affairs (Oceans and Coasts), Medical Research Council, Rhodes University and the University of the Western Cape.

Conflicts of Interest: The authors declare no conflict of interest.

References

1. Davies-Coleman, M.T.; Beukes, D.R. Ten years of marine natural products research at Rhodes University. *South Afr. J. Sci.* **2004**, *100*, 539–543. [CrossRef]
2. Davies-Coleman, M.T. Bioactive natural products from southern African marine invertebrates. In *Studies in Natural Product Chemistry (Bioactive Natural Products Part L)*; Atta-ur-Rahman, Ed.; Elsevier: Amsterdam, The Netherlands, 2005; Volume 32, pp. 61–107.
3. Sunassee, S.N.; Davies-Coleman, M.T. Marine bioprospecting in southern Africa. In *Drug Discovery in Africa*; Chibale, K., Masimbirembwe, C., Davies-Coleman, M., Eds.; Springer-Verlag: Heidelberg, Germany, 2012; pp. 193–210.
4. Proksch, P.; Edrada-Ebel, R.; Ebel, R. Drugs from the sea—Opportunities and obstacles. *Mar. Drugs* **2003**, *1*, 5–17. [CrossRef]
5. Pettit, G.R.; Inoue, M.; Kamano, Y.; Herald, D.L.; Arm, C.; Dufresne, C.; Christie, N.D.; Schmidt, J.M.; Doubek, D.L.; Krupa, T.S. Antineoplastic agents. 147. Isolation and structure of the powerful cell growth inhibitor cephalostatin 1. *J. Am. Chem. Soc.* **1988**, *110*, 2006–2007. [CrossRef]
6. Iglesias-Arteaga, M.A.; Morzycki, J.W. Cephalostatins and ritterazines. In *The Alkaloids: Chemistry and Biology*; Knölker, H.-J., Ed.; Academic Press: London, UK, 2013; Volume 72, pp. 153–279.
7. Rudy, A.; López-Antón, N.; Dirsch, V.M.; Vollmar, A.M. The cephalostatin way of apoptosis. *J. Nat. Prod.* **2008**, *71*, 482–486. [CrossRef] [PubMed]
8. Zhou, B.-N.; Hoch, J.M.; Johnson, R.K.; Mattern, M.R.; Eng, W.-K.; Ma, J.; Hecht, S.M.; Newman, D.J.; Kingston, D.G.I. Use of COMPARE analysis to discover new natural product drugs: Isolation of camptothecin and 9-methoxycamptothecin from a new source. *J. Nat. Prod.* **2000**, *63*, 1273–1276. [CrossRef] [PubMed]
9. Von Schwarzenberg, K.; Vollmar, A.M. Targeting apoptosis pathways by natural compounds in cancer: Marine compounds as lead structures and chemical tools for cancer therapy. *Cancer Lett.* **2013**, *332*, 295–303. [CrossRef] [PubMed]
10. Dirsch, V.M.; Müller, I.M.; Eichhorst, S.T.; Pettit, G.R.; Kamano, Y.; Inoue, M.; Xu, J.-P.; Ichihara, Y.; Wanner, G.; Vollmar, A.M. Cephalostatin 1 selectively triggers the release of Smac/DIABLO and subsequent apoptosis that is characterized by an increased density of the mitochondrial matrix. *Cancer Res.* **2003**, *63*, 8896–8876.
11. Burgett, A.W.G.; Poulsen, T.B.; Wangkanont, K.; Anderson, D.R.; Kikuchi, C.; Shimada, K.; Okubo, S.; Fortner, K.C.; Mimaki, Y.; Kuroda, M.; *et al.* Natural products reveal cancer cell dependence on oxysterol-binding proteins. *Nat. Chem. Biol.* **2011**, *7*, 639–647. [CrossRef]
12. Pettit, G.R.; Xu, J.P.; Chapuis, J.C.; Melody, N. The cephalostatins. 24. Isolation, structure, and cancer cell growth inhibition of cephalostatin 20. *J. Nat. Prod.* **2015**, *78*, 1446–1450. [CrossRef]
13. Fortner, K.C.; Kato, D.; Tanaka, Y.; Shair, M.D. Enantioselective synthesis of (+)-cephalostatin 1. *J. Am. Chem. Soc.* **2010**, *132*, 275–280. [CrossRef] [PubMed]
14. Shi, Y.; Jia, L.; Xiao, Q.; Lan, Q.; Tang, X.; Wang, D.; Li, M.; Ji, Y.; Zhou, T.; Tian, W. A practical synthesis of cephalostatin 1. *Chem. Asian J.* **2011**, *6*, 786–790. [CrossRef] [PubMed]
15. LaCour, T.G.; Guo, C.; Bhandaru, S.; Boyd, M.R.; Fuchs, P.L. Interphylal product splicing: The first total syntheses of cephalostatin 1, the north hemisphere of ritterazine G, and the highly active hybrid analogue, ritterostatin $G_N1_N{}^1$. *J. Am. Chem. Soc.* **1998**, *120*, 692–707. [CrossRef]

16. Kanduluru, A.K.; Banerjee, P.; Beutler, J.A.; Fuchs, P.L. A convergent total synthesis of the potent cephalostatin/ritterazine hybrid-25-*epi* ritterostatin G_N1_N. *J. Org. Chem.* **2013**, *78*, 9085–9092. [CrossRef] [PubMed]
17. Pettit, G.R.; Moser, B.R.; Herald, D.L.; Knight, J.C.; Chapuis, J.C.; Zheng, X. The cephalostatins. 23. Conversion of hecogenin to a steroidal 1,6-dioxaspiro[5.5]nonane analogue for cephalostatin 11. *J. Nat. Prod.* **2015**, *78*, 1067–1072. [CrossRef] [PubMed]
18. Sikorska, J.; Hau, A.M.; Anklin, C.; Parker-Nance, S.; Davies-Coleman, M.T.; Ishmael, J.E.; McPhail, K.L. Mandelalides A–D, cytotoxic macrolides from a new *Lissoclinum* species of South African tunicate. *J. Org. Chem.* **2012**, *77*, 6066–6075. [CrossRef]
19. Lei, H.; Yan, J.; Yu, J.; Liu, Y.; Wang, Z.; Xu, Z.; Ye, T. Total synthesis and stereochemical reassignment of mandelalide A. *Angew. Chem. Int. Ed.* **2014**, *53*, 6533–6537. [CrossRef]
20. Willwacher, J.; Heggen, B.; Wirtz, C.; Thiel, W.; Fürstner, A. Total synthesis, stereochemical revision, and biological reassessment of mandelalide A: Chemical mimicry of intrafamily relationships. *Chem. Eur. J.* **2015**, *21*, 10416–10430. [CrossRef] [PubMed]
21. Willwacher, J.; Fürstner, A. Catalysis-based total synthesis of putative mandelalide A. *Angew. Chem. Int. Ed.* **2014**, *53*, 4217–4221. [CrossRef] [PubMed]
22. Winder, P.L. Therapeutic Potential, Mechanism of Action, and Ecology of Novel Marine Natural Products. Ph.D. Thesis, Florida Atlantic University, Boca Raton, FL, USA, 2009.
23. Paterson, I.; Haslett, G.W. Synthesis of the C1–C11 western fragment of madeirolide A. *Org. Lett.* **2013**, *15*, 1338–1341. [CrossRef] [PubMed]
24. Reddy, K.M.; Yamini, V.; Singarapu, K.K.; Ghosh, S. Synthesis of proposed aglycone of mandelalide A. *Org. Lett.* **2014**, *16*, 2658–2660. [CrossRef] [PubMed]
25. Hiramatsu, K.; Cui, L.; Kuroda, M.; Ito, T. The emergence and evolution of methicillin-resistant *Staphylococcus aureus*. *Trends Microbiol.* **2001**, *9*, 486–493. [CrossRef]
26. Alanis, A.J. Resistance to antibiotics: Are we in the post-antibiotic era? *Arch. Med. Res.* **2005**, *36*, 697–705. [CrossRef] [PubMed]
27. Mole, B. Farming up trouble. *Nature* **2013**, *499*, 398–400. [CrossRef] [PubMed]
28. Fortuin-de Smidt, M.C.; Singh-Moodley, A.; Badat, R.; Quan, V.; Kularatne, R.; Nana, T.; Lekalakala, R.; Govender, N.P.; Perovic, O. *Staphylococcus aureus* bacteraemia in Gauteng academic hospitals, South Africa. *Int. J. Infect. Dis.* **2015**, *30*, 41–48. [CrossRef]
29. Lewis, K. Platforms for antibiotic discovery. *Nat. Rev. Drug Discov.* **2013**, *12*, 371–387. [CrossRef] [PubMed]
30. Zoraghi, R.; See, R.H.; Axerio-Cilies, P.; Kumar, N.S.; Gong, H.; Moreau, A.; Hsing, M.; Kaur, S.; Swayze, R.D.; Worrall, L.; *et al.* Identification of pyruvate kinase in methicillin-resistant *Staphylococcus aureus* as a novel antimicrobial drug target. *Antimicrob. Agents Chemother.* **2011**, *55*, 2042–2053. [CrossRef] [PubMed]
31. Cherkasov, A.; Hsing, M.; Zoraghi, R.; Foster, L.J.; See, R.H.; Stoynov, N.; Jiang, J.; Kaur, S.; Lian, T.; Jackson, L.; *et al.* Mapping the protein interaction network in methicillin-resistant *Staphylococcus aureus*. *J. Proteome Res.* **2011**, *10*, 1139–1150. [CrossRef] [PubMed]
32. Zoraghi, R.; Reiner, N.E. Protein interaction networks as starting points to identify novel antimicrobial drug targets. *Curr. Opin. Microbiol.* **2013**, *16*, 566–572. [CrossRef] [PubMed]
33. Kumar, N.S.; Amandoron, E.A.; Cherkasov, A.; Brett Finlay, B.; Gong, H.; Jackson, L.; Kaur, S.; Lian, T.; Moreau, A.; Labrière, C.; *et al.* Optimization and structure-activity relationships of a series of potent inhibitors of methicillin-resistant *Staphylococcus aureus* (MRSA) pyruvate kinase as novel antimicrobial agents. *Bioorg. Med. Chem.* **2012**, *20*, 7069–7082. [CrossRef]
34. Zoraghi, R.; Worrall, L.; See, R.H.; Strangman, W.; Popplewell, W.L.; Gong, H.; Samaai, T.; Swayze, R.D.; Kaur, S.; Vuckovic, M.; *et al.* Methicillin-resistant *Staphylococcus aureus* (MRSA) pyruvate kinase as a target for bis-indole alkaloids with antibacterial activities. *J. Biol. Chem.* **2011**, *286*, 44716–44725. [CrossRef] [PubMed]
35. Veale, C.G.L.; Zoraghi, R.; Young, R.M.; Morrison, J.P.; Pretheeban, M.; Lobb, K.A.; Reiner, N.E.; Andersen, R.J.; Davies-Coleman, M.T. Synthetic analogues of the marine bisindole deoxytopsentin: Potent selective inhibitors of MRSA pyruvate kinase. *J. Nat. Prod.* **2015**, *78*, 355–362. [CrossRef]
36. Veale, C.G.L.; Lobb, K.A.; Zoraghi, R.; Morrison, J.P.; Reiner, N.E.; Andersen, R.J.; Davies-Coleman, M.T. Synthesis and MRSA PK inhibitory activity of thiazole containing deoxytopsentin analogues. *Tetrahedron* **2014**, *70*, 7845–7853. [CrossRef]

37. Zoraghi, R.; Campbell, S.; Kim, C.; Dullaghan, E.M.; Blair, L.M.; Gillard, R.M.; Reiner, N.E.; Sperry, J. Discovery of a 1,2-bis(3-indolyl)ethane that selectively inhibits the pyruvate kinase of methicillin-resistant *Staphylococcus aureus* over human isoforms. *Bioorg. Med. Chem. Lett.* **2014**, *24*, 5059–5062. [CrossRef] [PubMed]
38. Blair, L.M.; Sperry, J. Palladium-catalyzed heteroannulation approach to 1,2-bis(3-indolyl)ethanes. *Synlett* **2013**, *24*, 1931–1936.
39. Kumar, N.S.; Dullaghan, E.M.; Finlay, B.B.; Gong, H.; Reiner, N.E.; Jon Paul Selvam, J.; Thorson, L.M.; Campbell, S.; Vitko, N.; Richardson, A.R.; *et al.* Discovery and optimization of a new class of pyruvate kinase inhibitors as potential therapeutics for the treatment of methicillin-resistant *Staphylococcus aureus* infections. *Bioorg. Med. Chem.* **2014**, *22*, 1708–1725. [CrossRef]

marine drugs

Review

Natural Product Research in the Australian Marine Invertebrate *Dicathais orbita*

Kirsten Benkendorff

Marine Ecology Research Center, School of Environment, Science and Engineering, Southern Cross University, PO Box 157, Lismore, NSW 2480, Australia; Kirsten.benkendorff@scu.edu.au; Tel.: +61-2-66203755; Fax: +61-2-66212669

Received: 14 January 2013; in revised form: 4 March 2013; Accepted: 8 March 2013; Published: 23 April 2013

Abstract: The predatory marine gastropod *Dicathais orbita* has been the subject of a significant amount of biological and chemical research over the past five decades. Natural products research on *D. orbita* includes the isolation and identification of brominated indoles and choline esters as precursors of Tyrian purple, as well as the synthesis of structural analogues, bioactivity testing, biodistributional and biosynthetic studies. Here I also report on how well these compounds conform to Lipinski's rule of five for druglikeness and their predicted receptor binding and enzyme inhibitor activity. The composition of mycosporine-like amino acids, fatty acids and sterols has also been described in the egg masses of *D. orbita*. The combination of bioactive compounds produced by *D. orbita* is of interest for further studies in chemical ecology, as well as for future nutraceutical development. Biological insights into the life history of this species, as well as ongoing research on the gene expression, microbial symbionts and biosynthetic capabilities, should facilitate sustainable production of the bioactive compounds. Knowledge of the phylogeny of *D. orbita* provides an excellent platform for novel research into the evolution of brominated secondary metabolites in marine molluscs. The range of polarities in the brominated indoles produced by *D. orbita* has also provided an effective model system used to develop a new method for biodistributional studies. The well characterized suite of chemical reactions that generate Tyrian purple, coupled with an in depth knowledge of the ecology, anatomy and genetics of *D. orbita* provide a good foundation for ongoing natural products research.

Keywords: bioactivity; biosynthesis; brominated secondary metabolites; choline ester; indole

1. Introduction

Dicathais orbita, commonly known as the Australian Dogwhelk or Cartrut shell, is a predatory marine gastropod in the family Muricidae. This family of marine molluscs is well known for the production of the ancient dye Tyrian purple [1,2], which was the first marine natural product to be structurally elucidated by Friedlander in 1909 [3]. Over a century later, there remain major gaps in our knowledge of the ecological role and biosynthesis of this secondary metabolite [4,5]. However, significant progress has been made by Australian researchers over the last five decades [1,6–15], thus providing a foundation for using *D. orbita* as model species in natural products research.

As a common and relatively large gastropod on rocky intertidal reefs, *Dicathais orbita* is an important educational resource and has been the focus of study by a wide diversity of Australian postgraduate research students. Investigations into the natural products of *D. orbita* first commenced with the Ph.D. thesis of Joe Baker in 1967 [9], who established the ultimate precursors of Tyrian purple from the biosynthetic organ, the hypobranchial gland (e.g., Figure 1). This work was continued in the Ph.D. thesis of Colin Duke [16], who identified the intermediate precursors and synthesized a range of structural analogues. After a twenty year gap, my Ph.D. study into the antimicrobial properties of Australian molluskan egg masses identified the precursors of Tyrian purple from *D. orbita* as interesting lead compounds for bioactivity studies [17]. This initiated an ongoing program of research focused on *D. orbita* and their bioactive compounds, resulting in the completion of a further four Ph.D.s [18–21], one Masters of Biotechnology [22] and eight Honors theses [23–30], with an additional five Ph.D.s currently in progress.

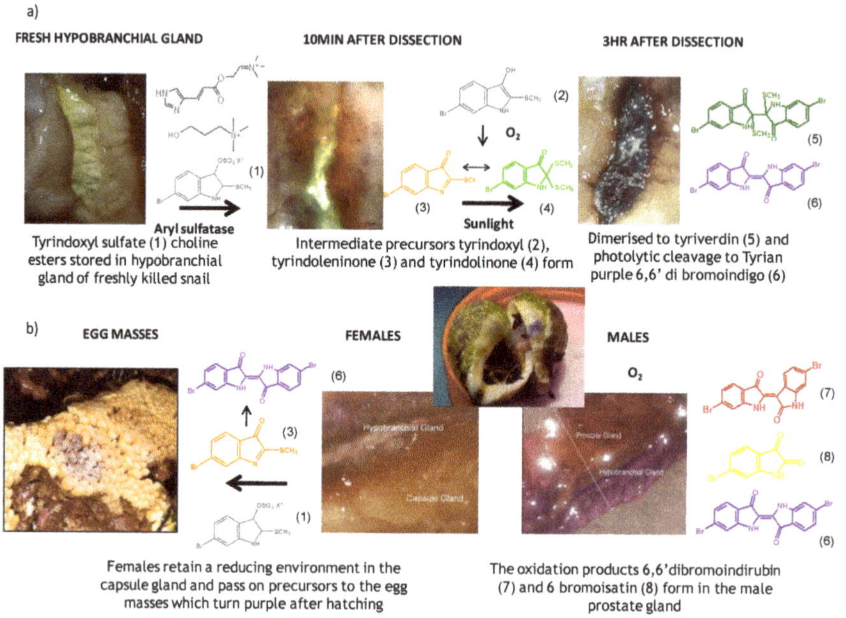

Figure 1. (**a**) The development of Tyrian purple in the hypobranchial gland of *Dicathais orbita*; (**b**) The transfer of reduced precursors from the capsule gland of females to the egg capsules and the oxidation of precursors in the prostate gland of male *D. orbita*.

Around the same time as the research on *D. orbita* natural products chemistry commenced, Australia research students began investigating the ecology and life history of this species. The first in-depth study into the biology of *D. (aegrota) orbita* was undertaken by Bruce Phillips in Western Australia, whose Ph.D. thesis was published in 1968 [31]. Several additional student theses investigating the life history and ecology of *D. orbita* have been recently undertaken in South Australia [24,28,29]. *Dicathais (Thais) orbita* was also the major focus of a Ph.D. thesis by Gibson investigating imposex caused by TBT pollution on the east coast of Australia [32]. This established *D. orbita* as one of the first Australian invertebrate model species for ecotoxicology and an important indicator for environmental monitoring [32]. *D. orbita* was also included in the Ph.D. thesis of well known Australian ecologist Peter Fairweather, who investigated interactions between predators and prey on intertidal shores [33]. *D. orbita* has been subsequently included as a model species in several other student theses investigating environmental stressors and human impacts [34,35]. These insights into the ecology and life history of *D. orbita* have greatly facilitated ongoing natural products research, through interesting biological insights and population assessments, which help ensure sustainable collection.

To be suitable as a model system for innovative natural products chemistry research, a wealth of biological data is required on the organism, along with extensive familiarity with secondary metabolism system to be studied. *Dicathais orbita* is a candidate model species for the biosynthesis of brominated indoles, as these natural products and the associated biosynthetic glands in this marine mollusk are relatively well known (Figure 1). Useful biological traits for the selection of model species also include availability and life history features that make them easy to manipulate and maintain in the laboratory, as well as genetic knowledge and potential economic benefit [36]. Indeed *D. orbita* is a relatively large, long-lived gastropod that is common on rocky reefs in temperature Australian waters [33,37–39] and it also occurs as a pest predator on some molluskan aquaculture farms [40]. This species produces benthic egg capsules that each contain thousands of embryos that can be studied through several stages of larval development [41] and the reproductive cycle and anatomy of the adults is well documented [15,42,43]. *D. orbita* is resilient to environmental fluctuations [pers. obs] and both broodstock and juveniles can be easily maintained in laboratory aquaria [44]. The taxonomy of this species is well resolved [45], as is its systematic position within the Rapaninae subfamily of Muricidae [46] and the Gastropoda [47–49] more broadly. Genetic information on this species is also accumulating [5,50], with preliminary genome sequencing currently underway. A significant transcriptome database exists for a related species of *Rapaninae* [51]. As highlighted by Rittschof, and McClellan-Green [36], the power of model organisms could increase exponentially with input from multidisciplinary research teams that work from the molecular level, through the various levels of biological organization, to the ecosystem level. The combination of natural products chemistry and biological research undertaken on *D. orbita* to date establishes this species as potentially useful model for future studies on the evolution and biosynthesis of marine secondary metabolites, as well as for new method development e.g., [52].

2. Secondary Metabolites from *Dicathais orbita*

2.1. Brominated Indole Derivatives

The hypobranchial gland of muricid mollusks is the source of the ancient dye Tyrian purple, for which the main pigment is well established to be a brominated derivative of indole, 6,6 dibromoindigo (**6**, Figure 1) [1–3]. Original observations of the hypobranchial glands confirmed that the dye pigment itself is not present in the live mollusk, but rather is generated after a series of enzymatic, oxidative and photolytic reactions. In 1685, Cole [53] first described the changes in the hypobranchial glands of muricid mollusks, from a white fluid to yellow, through various shades of green and blue, before obtaining the final purple color after exposure to sunlight. This series of color reactions was also noted by Baker [1,8,9] in the hypobranchial glands from the Australian species *D. orbita*; illustrated in Figure 1. The indole precursors span a range of chemical properties (Table 1a) from the water soluble salt of tyrindoxyl sulfate (M.W. 337, 339, log $p < -0.3$) to the highly insoluble tyriverdin (M.W. 514, 516, 518, log $p > 4.6$).

Baker and Sutherland [8] first isolated a salt of tyrindoxyl sulphate (**1**, Figure 1) from an ethanol extract of the hypobranchial gland of *D. orbita* and identified this as the ultimate precursor to the dye Tyrian purple. They also isolated an enzyme with sulfatase activity capable of hydrolyzing tyrindoxyl sulfate and initiating the production of Tyrian purple by exposure to sunlight [8]. Baker and Duke [6,7,10,11] subsequently isolated and identified the intermediate precursors tyrindoxyl (**2**) and tyrindoleninone (6-bromo-2-methylthio-3*H*-indol-3-one) (**3**), as well as tyrindolinone (**4**), a methanethiol adduct of tyrindoleninone (Figure 1a). Using various organic solvents, Baker and Sutherland were also able to isolate a yellow light insensitive compound identified as 6-bromoisatin, and the immediate precursor to Tyrian purple, a green light sensitive compound tyriverdin [8]. The structure of tyriverdin (**5**, Figure 1) was subsequently corrected by Christophersen *et al.* [54] as an indole dimer that forms spontaneously from the reaction between tyrindoxyl and tyrindoleninone (Figure 1a). 6-Bromoisatin (**8**, Figure 1) is considered to be an oxidation artifact in this sequence of reactions [2,8] and is a precursor of the red Tyrian purple isomer 6,6′-dibromoindirubin (**7**) [55]. These oxidation products do occur naturally in small amounts of the extracts from males, but were not detected in female *D. orbita* hyprobranchial gland and gonad extracts (Figure 1b), suggesting sex specific differences in the chemical environment of these glands [13].

Table 1. Molecular properties of (**A**) brominated indoles and (**B**) choline esters isolated from *Dicathais orbita* using Molinspiration Cheminformatics (2012). Molecular weight for Br^{79} isotopes.

Compound	MW/Formula	Log *p* [a]	Polar surface area/volume	No. non-H atoms	No. H bond acceptors [b]	No. H bond donors [c]	Rotatable bonds	No. rule of 5 violations [d]
Tyrindoxyl sulfate 	337.196 $C_9H_7BrNO_4S_2^-$	−0.346	82.224/211.287	17	5	1	3	0
Tyrindoxyl	258.14 C_9H_8BrNOS	3.375	36.019/173.614	13	2	2	1	0
6 Bromoisatin 	226.029 C_8H_4BrNOS	1.615	49.933/141.457	12	3	1	0	0
Tyrindoleninone	256.124 C_9H_6BrNOS	2.889	29.963/168.021	13	2	0	1	0
Tyrindolinone	304.234 $C_{10}H_{10}BrNOS_2$	2.999	29.098/208.356	15	2	1	2	0
Tyriverdin 	514.264 $C_{18}H_{14}Br_2N_2O_2S_2$	4.66	58.196/334.697	26	4	2	3	1
Tyrian purple 6,6′ dibromoindigo 	420.06 $C_{16}H_8Br_2N_2O_2$	4.47	65.724/259.728	22	4	2	0	0
6,6′ Dibromoindirubin 	420.06 $C_{16}H_8Br_2N_2O_2$	4.47	65.724/259.728	22	4	2	0	0

(**A**)

Compound	MW/Formula	Log *p* [a]	Polar surface area/volume	No. non-H atoms	No. H bond acceptors [b]	No. H bond donors [c]	Rotatable bonds	No. rule of 5 violations [d]
Murexine 	224.284 $C_{11}H_{18}N_3O_2^+$	−3.373	54.988/219.763	16	5	1	5	0
Senecoiycholine 	186.275 $C_{10}H_{20}NO_2^+$	−2.096	26.305/200.647	13	3	0	5	0
Tigloylcholine 	186.275 $C_{10}H_{20}NO_2^+$	−2.33	26.305/200.647	13	3	0	5	0
Choline	104.173 $C_5H_{14}NO^+$	−4.236	20.228/120.158	7	2	1	2	0

(**B**)

[a] Log *p* is based on octanol-water partition coefficient; [b] H bond acceptors include O & N atoms; [c] H bond donors include OH and NH groups; [d] Rule of 5 violations are based on the molecular descriptors used by Lipinski *et al.* [56] for "drug-like" molecules (log $p \leq 5$, molecular weight ≤ 500, number of hydrogen bond acceptors ≤ 10, and number of hydrogen bond donors ≤ 5).

An interesting point of difference in *D. orbita* indole chemistry, relative to other Muricidae, is the production of a single brominated ultimate precursor molecule [2,8,57]. Four prochromogens including brominated and nonbrominated indoxyl sulfates have been suggested for *Murex brandaris* [58], which then generate a mixture of purple 6,6 dibromoindigo, as well as blue indigo and monobromoindigo [2]. Baker [1] also demonstrated the complexity of purple precursors obtained from the hypobranchial glands of some other Muricidae species. These Tyrian purple precursors are also transferred to the egg masses of *D. orbita* (Figure 1b) and other Muricidae mollusks [12,59]. Similar to the hypobranchial glands, the egg masses of other Muricidae were found to contain a more complex mixture of brominated and non brominated indole, as well as other brominated compounds including imidazoles, quinolones and quinoxalines [17,60,61]. Consequently, the Australian species *D. orbita* appears to be a particularly pure source of 6,6′ dibromoindigo and the simplicity of the single precursor make it a good model for biosynthetic studies of brominated indoles. On the other hand, the diversity of indoles and brominated compounds in the Muricidae family more broadly provides a good opportunity for phylogenetic investigations into the evolution of secondary metabolism.

2.2. Choline Esters

In 1976, Baker and Duke made an important breakthrough when they isolated choline from the hypobranchial glands of *D. orbita* and demonstrated that tyrindoxyl sulfate is stored as a choline ester salt [7]. This salt is hydrolysed by an arylsulphatase enzyme, which is also stored within the hypobranchial gland [8], to generate the intermediate precursors of Tyrian purple (Figure 1a). Both choline, and to a lesser extent murexine (β-imidazolyl-4(5)acrylcholine) (Table 1b) were found to be associated with tyrindoxyl sulfate [7]. *N*-Methylmurexine was also suggested to be present in the hypobranchial gland extracts [7], but this was subsequently questioned by Duke *et al.* [62,63].

In 1996, Roseghini *et al.* [64] reported a survey of choline esters and biogenic amines from the hypobranchial glands of 55 species of gastropods. *Dicathais* (*Neothais*) *orbita* was found to contain significant quantities of murexine and senecioylcholine (Table 1b). Dihydromurexine was the dominant choline ester found in some other Muricidae species, but was not detected in *D. orbita* [64]. Shiomi *et al.* [65] have also identified tigloylcholine (Table 1b) in other muricids from the genus *Thais*. These authors pointed out that senecioylcholine is a structural isomer of tigloylcholine and since senecioylcholine was only previously identified by thin layer chromatography and is indistinguishable from tigloylcholine using this method, it may have been misidentified in the earlier studies [65].

2.3. Mycosporine-Like Amino Acids, Fatty Acids and Sterols in the Egg Masses

In addition to reports on the indole derivatives in *D. orbita* egg masses [60,66], the composition of mycosporine-like amino acids (MAAs) and fatty acids has been documented for this species. MAAs are small sunscreening compounds with an absorption maxima of 310–360 nm [67]. They are produced via the shikimate pathway in algae, fungi and bacteria, but animals, including marine invertebrates, are thought to acquire these secondary metabolites through diet or symbiosis [67,68]. Przeslawski *et al.* [69] revealed that mycosporine-glycine and shinorine were the dominant MAAs in *D. orbita*, along with porphyra-334 and mycosporine-2-glycine and trace amounts of palythine. Mycosporine-taurine, palythene, asterina-330 and palythinol were not detected in this species, although an additional unknown peak with an absorption maxima of λ 307 nm was reported in *D. orbita*, along with two other Muricidae [69]. The composition of MAAs was found to be strongly influenced by phylogeny in molluskan egg masses, but not by the adult diet or levels of UV exposure in the spawning habitat [69]. This suggests that predatory marine mollusks, such as *D. orbita*, are able to bioaccumulate MAAs from their prey and transfer these into the egg masses to protect their developing embryos. Higher MAA concentrations were found in *D. orbita* egg masses with viable embryos in comparison to inviable egg masses [69]. The inviable eggs of *D. orbita* typically appear pink or purple in color, as opposed to the usual yellow color [59], thus indicating further chemical changes, likely due to the photolytic degradation of Tyrian purple precursors. By absorbing UV radiation in normally developing Muricidae egg masses, MAAs may play an essential role in maintaining the bioactive indole precursors prior to larval hatching. Alternatively, by absorbing in the UV spectra [13,27], the brominated indoles may provide further protection against harmful UV rays.

In a comparative study of lipophylic extracts of the egg masses from a range of molluskan species, Benkendorff *et al.* [70] revealed that *D. orbita* egg capsules predominately contain palmitic and stearic acid. Unlike many other gastropod egg masses, no unsaturated fatty acids were found in the leathery egg capsules of *D. orbita* and related neogastropods [70]. The extracts from *D. orbita* egg masses contained a large amount of sterol, predominately cholesterol, but with smaller amounts of cholestadienol, cholestanol, methyl cholestadienol and methylcholestenol [70]. No cholestadiene or stigmatenone were found, although some unknown sterols were detected. It is unclear why Neogastropoda with leathery egg capsules, such as *D. orbita*, have a much higher saturated fatty acid and sterol content than gastropods with gelatinous egg masses, although the later may require unsaturated fatty acids to maintain fluidity in the gelatinous matrix.

3. Bioactivity of *Dicathais orbita* Extracts and Compounds

3.1. *Drug-Likeness of* D. orbita *Secondary Metabolites*

Using the online chemoinformatics software Molinspiration (version 2011.06) the drug-likeness (Table 1) and bioactivity scores (Table 2) are predicted for the main secondary metabolites from *D. orbita*. Drug-likeness is based on Lipinskis "Rule of 5" [69], which considers whether various molecular properties and structure features of a particular molecule are similar to known drugs. These properties, such as hydrophobicity, electronic distribution, hydrogen bonding characteristics, molecule size and flexibility (Table 2), influence the bioavailability, transport properties, affinity to proteins, reactivity, toxicity, metabolic stability of the molecule and thus potential for use as a pharmaceutical drug. Of all the indole derivatives examined (Table 1a), only a single violation of the rule of 5 was found. This was for tyriverdin, due to a molecule weight exceeding 500 mass units (Table 1a). As expected, choline and all of the choline esters conform to the rule of 5 for drug-likeness (Table 1b).

Table 2. Bioactivity of (**A**) brominated indoles and (**B**) choline esters isolated from *Dicathais orbita* based on calculated distribution of activity scores from Molinspiration (version 2011.06) #, as well as known bioactivity from the published literature.

Compound	GPCR ligand	Ion channel modulator	Kinase inhibitor	Nuclear receptor ligand	Protease inhibitor	Enzyme inhibitor	Other known bioactivity
Tyrindoxyl sulfate 	0.22 *	0.02	−0.13	−0.36	0.10	0.73 **	-
Tyrindoxyl	−0.56	−0.09	−0.41	−0.71	−1.00	−0.11	Unstable in O_2
6 Bromoisatin 	−1.08	−0.49	0.50	−1.62	−1.07	−0.39	Anticancer, induces apoptosis, anti-bacterial [12,71]
Tyrindoleninone	−0.93	−0.39	−0.69	−1.16	−1.15	−0.43	Anticancer, induces apoptosis, anti-bacterial [12,71]
Tyrindolinone	−0.87	−0.54	−0.89	−1.03	−0.93	−0.51	Unstable in O_2
Tyriverdin 	−0.23	−0.23	−0.29	−0.34	−0.17	−0.17	Bacteriostatic, inhibits FDA hydrolysis [12]
Tyrian purple 6,6′ Dibromoindigo 	−0.32	−0.30	0.22 *	−0.05	−0.36	−0.01	Highly insoluble, no apparent antibacterial or anticancer activity [4]
6,6′ Dibromoindirubin 	−0.78	−0.74	0.45 *	−0.28	−0.61	0.01	GSK-3 inhibitor [72]

(**A**)

Compound	GPCR ligand	Ion channel modulator	Kinase inhibitor	Nuclear receptor ligand	Protease inhibitor	Enzyme inhibitor	Other known bioactivity
Murexine 	0.38 *	0.50 *	−0.16	−1.70	−0.36	0.84 **	Neuromuscular blocking and nicotinic action. No muscarinic effects. Paralysis of the skeletal musculature, toxic to mice at high doses (i.v. LD_{50} 8.5 mg/kg, s.c. LD_{50} = 50 mg/kg); human clinical dose (EC_{50} = 1 mg/kg) [63,73]
Senecioylcholine 	−0.39	0.33 *	−1.04	−1.28	−0.95	0.35 *	Neuromuscular blocking and nicotinic action. No muscarinic effects [63]
Tigloylcholine 	−0.45	0.32 *	−1.37	−1.31	−1.35	0.41 *	Toxic to mice (i.v. LD_{50} = 0.92 mg/kg) [64]
Choline 	−2.64	−2.21	−3.84	−4.93	−3.94	−2.18	Essential nutrient, precursor for the neurotransmitter acetyl choline [74]

(**B**) # Larger value bioactivity scores indicate a higher probability that the molecule will be active; * potential activity; ** high potential activity.

The drug-likeness for Tyrian purple maybe over-estimated. The log *p* values for 6,6-dibromoindigo is perhaps lower than anticipated considering the fact that this compound is highly non-polar and generally insoluble at room temperature in all organic solvents [2]. Tyrian purple can only be extracted out of tissue or cloth using hot (>100 °C) DMF or DMSO. It appears to form dimers or higher polymers due to the van der Waals attraction between bromine atoms [75], which contribute to the high stability of the compound, but nevertheless the low solubility makes it an unlikely drug candidate. Despite the same log *p* value (Table 1a) 6,6′ dibromoindirubin appears to be slightly more soluble in non-polar solvents at room temperature (pers. obs.), perhaps due to reduced polymer formation in this isomer.

3.2. *Bioactivity of* D. orbita *Brominated Indoles*

The predicted Molinspiration bioactivity scores for *D. orbita* brominated indoles identify the ultimate precursor tyrindoxyl sulfate as the most likely pharmacophore. This compound shows potential as a GPCR ligand and enzyme inhibitor (Table 2a). Unlike the intermediate precursor compounds, this polar brominated indoxyl sulfate salt has not been directly tested for cytotoxicity in antibacterial and anticancer screening assays. This is because bioassay guided fractionation of *D. orbita* extracts has revealed most of the activity in the more lipophilic fractions of chloroform extracts and generally no activity is found in the polar methanol water fractions [12,19,26,71,76,77], where tyrindoxyl sulfate is mostly concentrated. Nevertheless, tyrindoxyl sulfate has been present in some of the anticancer extracts showing bioactivity against MCF-7 breast cancer cells *in vitro* [26] and against DNA damaged colon cells *in vivo* [78] and could contribute to the observed activity. Tyrindoxyl sulfate is likely to be metabolized and transported differently to the other less polar compounds *in vivo* (Table 1a). This, along with the predicted enzyme binding activity, suggests that tyrindoxyl sulfate might be worthy of further bioactivity studies.

At the other extreme of polarity (Table 1a), the Tyrian purple pigments have predicted protein kinase receptor interaction (Table 1b). This predicted activity is supported for 6,6′ dibromoindirubin, which was shown to be a selective GSK-3 inhibitor, but with limited activity against CDK1/Cyclin B or CDK5/p25 [72,79]. The 6,6′ dibromoindigo isomer was not tested in this study and although predicted to have some protein kinase activity (Table 2a), the extreme insolubility of this compound presents problems for bioactivity assessment.

Despite the compatibility with drug-likeness, few of the intermediate brominated indoles from *D. orbita* produced high enough bioactivity scores on Molinspiration to indicate interesting pharmacophores for receptor binding (Table 2a). Nevertheless, purified extracts containing 6-bromoisatin and tyrindoleninone do show broad spectrum antibacterial and anticancer activities [4,12,19,23,71,77,80]. Of particular interest is the >100 fold selective cytotoxicity towards human lymphoma and female reproductive cancer cell lines (KGN, JAr, OVCAR-3), compared to freshly isolated untransformed peripheral blood monocytes and female granulosa cells [19,22,23,71,80]. Furthermore, these brominated indole derivatives appear to induce apoptosis rather than necrosis in the reproductive cancer cell lines, as indicated by caspase 3/7 activity and DNA fragmentation from TUNNEL staining [19,71]. Preliminary work on these brominated indoles using flow cytometry with propidium iodine and annexin staining indicates they also induce apoptosis in lymphoma cells but not in $CaCO_2$ colon cancer cells [23,77,81]. However, more recent studies on purified 6-bromoisatin and tyrindoleninine indicate they do induce apoptosis in the H2T9 colon cancer cell line [81]. Furthermore, a rodent model for colon cancer using a concentrated extract containing these two brominated indoles shows that apoptosis is induced *in vivo* and unpublished studies indicate that 6-bromoisatin is the main active factor [81]. The mode of action for these brominated indole derivatives is currently unknown and as they are unlikely to bind with the receptors or enzymes listed in Table 2, further studies are required.

The dimeric compound tyriverdin was not predicted to have any bioactivity based on known pharmacophores for receptor or enzyme binding (Table 2a). Nevertheless, this compound has been identified as a potent bacteriostatic agent against a range of human and marine pathogens, using bioassay guided fractionation of *D. orbita* extracts with the flourescein diacetate hydrolysis antibacterial assay [12]. However, further testing of this compound with alternative methods, such as the standard plate dilution assay [12] or the MTS tetrazolium salt cell proliferation assay [26,27] has failed to confirm the antibacterial activity. Additional procedural controls have indicated that tyriverdin can partially quench the green fluorescence of flourescein in the absence of bacterial cells [27]. However, this quenching did not account for all the apparent reduction in fluorescein absorbance, suggesting that tyriverdin may also interfere with esterase activity or some other mechanism of converting flourescein diacetate to flourescien. However, in addition to violating the molecular weight rule for drug-likeness (Table 1a), tyriverdin also has solubility and instability problems. It is only slightly soluble in some solvents, such as chloroform and dichloromethane, but tends to precipitate out of most solvents (e.g., ether extracts [8] and toluene/hexane [27]), then decomposes to Tyrian purple. This low solubility along with its instability in sunlight and high molecular weight make it an unlikely drug-candidate.

3.3. Bioactivity of Choline Esters

Unlike the brominated indole derivatives, the choline esters naturally occurring in *D. orbita* obtained high bioactivity scores in the Molinspiration online chemoinformatics prediction software (Table 2b). In particular, all three choline esters were predicted to inhibit enzymes and modulate ion channels. Murexine, with an imidazole moiety, obtained the highest bioactivity scores and was also the only choline ester predicted to bind to GPCR (Table 2b). The prediction for ion channel modulation is consistent with the known biological activities of these choline esters. Murexine in particular has been thoroughly investigated for toxicity, paralysis of the skeletal musculature, neuromuscular blocking activity and nicotinic action [64,73,82,83] and similar pharmacological properties have been reported for senecioylcholine [64]. Both compounds are almost devoid of muscarinic effects on acetylcholine receptors [64,73]. Murexine was shown to stimulate ganglion, in addition to having depolarizing neuromuscular blocking actions in cat, dog and rat [82].

The intravenous LD_{50} for murexine in mice has been established at 6.5 mg/kg [64] to 8.7 mg/kg [73] and death is caused by anoxia secondary to peripheral respiratory arrest [64,73]. Tigloylcholine was estimated to be more toxic, with an i.v. LD_{50} of 0.92 mg/kg in mice [65]. When administered subcutaneously the LD_{50} of murexine in mice was approximately 50 mg/kg and oral delivery was ineffective in doses up to 1 g/kg [64]. Preliminary human clinical trials were conducted with murexine as muscle relaxant on 160 patients. The mean paralysing dose in adult patients was approximately 1 mg/kg i.v. with the paralysis lasting for 3–6 min after a single dose and longer lasting muscular relaxation could be obtained by slow i.v. infusion of a 1/1000 solution of murexine in physiological saline [64,73]. However, murexine caused several side-effects, which were mainly attributable to the nicotinic actions of the drug.

3.4. Antibacterial Activity and Chemical Ecology of the Egg Masses

As part of a screening study on the antimicrobial properties of molluskan egg masses, *Dicathais orbita* was identified as a species of particular interest, with the lipophylic extracts showing strong activity against a range of human and marine bacterial pathogens [66,84]. Bio-guided fractionation identified the brominated indole precursors of Tyrian purple as being responsible for this activity [12]. Based on this activity, Benkendorff *et al.* [12] proposed that defense of the developing embryos against ubiquitous marine pathogens could be the naturally selected role for these brominated indoles in Muricidae evolution. Consistent with this, the surface of the egg capsules of *D. orbita* were found to have very low levels of bacterial biofilm formation, with a high proportion of dead bacteria indicated by live/dead bacterial staining [85]. Using the MTS cell proliferation and broth dilution assay, extracts containing the Tyrian purple precursors from the surface of *D. orbita* egg capsules were effective at inhibiting the growth of the marine biofilm forming bacteria *Pseudoalteromonas* sp. S91, as well as the molluskan pathogen *Vibrio harveyi* [28]. The egg capsules of *D. orbita* were also found to have no protists on the surface and were relatively free of algal fouling compared to other gastropod egg masses [86]. The low surface fouling on these egg masses is likely to be due to a combination of chemical, physical and mechanical defense mechanisms preventing bacterial attachment and persistence on the surface [85].

To investigate whether fatty acids could contribute to the observed antibacterial activity in liphophylic extracts from mollusks [66,76], Benkendorff *et al.* [70] tested a series of lipid mixtures modeled on those found in the egg masses. The lipid mixture modeled on the fatty acid and sterol composition of *D. orbita* and similar Neogastropoda had very limited antibacterial activity against marine pathogens, especially when compared to species with gelatinous egg masses and a high content of polyunsaturated fatty acids [70]. It is possible that the bioactive indoles in *D. orbita* egg masses [12,60] negate the requirement for antimicrobial polyunsaturated fatty acids, or perhaps the transfer of bioactive indoles for defense of the egg masses was selected for due to the absence of alternative secondary metabolites with antibacterial activity in these egg masses.

3.5. Anti-Cancer Extracts, Toxicity & Nutraceutical Potential

Organic extracts from *D. orbita* egg masses, hypobranchial glands and mucus secretion effectively inhibit the proliferation of a range of cancer cell lines [19,23,26,71,77]. Bioassay guided fractionation indicated that the brominated indoles tyrindoleninone and tyrindolinone, as well as 6-bromoisatin are primarily responsible for this activity. A crude chloroform extract containing these brominated indole derivatives has also been shown to stimulate the acute apoptotic response to DNA-damage in the distal colon of mice, thus preventing early stage tumor formation [78]. Unpublished studies from my laboratory on the crude extracts and purified indoles suggest that these have no negative impacts on human immune cell function [22]. The crude extracts are generally not toxic in rodents, but can cause mild idiosyncratic hepatotoxicity in some mice [87]. Nevertheless, some liver damage is common with most chemotherapeutics and *D. orbita* extracts remain of interest due to their selective induction of apoptosis in cancerous or DNA damaged cells [71,78]. Further studies currently underway in my laboratory indicate that purified fractions containing the main active factor 6-bromoisatin have no effect on liver enzymes or hepatocytes *in vivo* [81]. As muricids comprise a traditional component of African [88], European [89], Mediterranean [90] and Asian [91] diets, there is excellent potential for the development of *D. orbita* as a novel medicinal food, particularly for colorectal cancer prevention, due to apparent bioavailability in the gastrointestinal tract. The historical and ongoing consumption of muricid meat implies an absence of symptomatic toxicity, although thorough investigation of the specific bioactive extracts is still required.

The combination of compounds with a range of bioactivities in the extracts of *D. orbita* is of particular interest for nutraceutical development [40,92]. In addition to the anticancer and antibacterial properties, *D. orbita* extracts appear to have a biphasic effect on progesterone steroidogenesis [19]. Furthermore, indirubin and some indoles are known to have anti-inflammatory properties. 5-Bromoisatin has been patented as an analgesic with sedative properties that reduce bleeding time in mice [93], suggesting 6-bromoisatin in *D. orbita* extracts could also have similar properties. To date, crude extracts from *D. orbita* containing choline esters not have been specifically tested for bioactivity or toxicity, despite the known muscle relaxing activity of these compounds (Table 2b). However, it is logical to assume than a concentrated extract containing these choline esters would retain the associated biological activity. Choline esters have also been suggested to act as immunological adjuvants in combined chemotherapy [94]. An extract containing muscle-relaxing, analgesic properties, antibacterial and anticancer activity could be particularly useful as a nutracetical or medicinal food [40]. Further studies are required to obtain an optimal concentration and combination of compounds to minimize any clinical side effects.

4. A Biological Basis for Future Natural Products Research

4.1. *Biosynthesis of* D. orbita *Brominated Indoles*

Basic gaps in our understanding of the gene and protein machinery that underlie Tyrian purple biosynthesis allow for new and exciting discoveries on biohalogenation and methane thiol incorporation into secondary metabolites. Tyrian purple is thought to be synthesized from dietary derived tryptophan in the Muricidae [4,43]. Tryptophan has been detected in the hypobranchial secretory cells of several Muricidae species [14,15]. It is particularly prevalent in the rectum of *D. orbita*, which is embedded in the hypobranchial gland [15,18]. Although it remains unclear how this amino acid is specifically converted into tyrindoxyl sulfate in Muricidae, several biosynthetic enzymes are likely to be involved (Table 3). Tryptophanase is typically involved in converting tryptophan to indole in bacteria, which can then be converted to indoxyl sulphate by a mono- or di-oxygenase enzyme system [95]. The specific enzymes involved in adding methane thiol groups onto the indole ring are unknown, but may involve some sulfur transferase and reductase enzymes (Table 3). Further investigation of these enzymes could uncover novel mechanisms for biotransformation in secondary metabolism.

Table 3. Biosynthetic enzymes proposed to be involved in the production of Tyrian purple precursors. The order of enzyme reactions generating the bromo and methylthio derivatives is not known.

Precursor/Substrate	Enzyme	Product
Tryptophan	Trytophanase	Indole
Indole	Dioxygenases	Indoxyl sulfate
Indole/Indoxyl sulfate	Bromoperoxidase	6 Bromoindole/Indoxyl
(6 Bromo) Indoxyl sulfate	Sulfur transferase & Sulfur reductase	(6 Bromo) Methylthio indolone/Tyrindoxyl sulfate
Tyrindoxyl sulfate	Aryl sulfatase	Tyrindoxyl

Specific incorporation of bromine into the 6-position of the indole ring is an unusual feature found in several bioactive marine indoles [96]. Since bromination more ready occurs in the 4 or 7 position, this strongly implies enzymatic bromination during the biosynthesis of tryindoxyl sulfate. Several regiospecific halogenases have been previously identified from bacteria, which are highly substrate specific for tryptophan [97,98]. However, the tryptophan-halogenases reported to date all appear to utilise chlorine over bromine. Jannun and Coe [99,100] reported bromoperoxidase activity in homogenates from hypobranchial glands of *Murex trunculus* and recent histochemical studies by Westley have confirmed the bromoperoxidase activity in *D. orbita* hypobranchial gland tissue [14,18]. A range of bromoperoxidase enzymes have been previously identified from marine algae, bacteria and fungi [101,102], but these do not generally appear to be substrate or regiospecific in their brominating activity. In a preliminary attempt to identify the bromoperoxidase gene from *D. orbita*, Laffy [21] developed primers from consensus sequence regions after multiple sequence alignment of 11 bromoperoxidases available on genebank (4 algal and 3 bacteria). No PCR products were amplified with these primers, despite successful positive controls. This indicates the muricid enzyme shares low sequence conservation at these primer sites or may be a distinct type of brominating enzyme with specificity for 6-bromination of tryptophan/indole for Tyrian purple biosynthesis. Bromination of indole derivatives has been shown to increase their biological activity [80,103] and the identification of novel halogenation strategies will facilitate alternative mechanisms for generating halogenated biologically active molecules for drug development [97].

The conversion of tyrindoxyl sulfate salt to tyrindoxyl and ultimately Tyrian purple requires an aryl sulfatase enzyme [8]. Histochemical studies have confirmed the release of aryl sulfatase on the epithelium of the hypobranchial gland of *D. orbita* [14,18]. Preliminary analysis of the transcriptome from *D. orbita* hypobranchial gland was successful in detecting the aryl sulfatase gene [5,21,50] and full length sequencing has confirmed the molluscan origin of this enzyme [21]. No other biosynthetic genes were identified in this mollusc transcriptome library, although there is good support for a primary role of the hypobranchial gland in protein synthesis, post translational modification and transport [5, 21,25,50]. A large number of unidentified sequences were also present in the hyporbanchial gland transcriptome, suggesting possible novel genes, although the suppressive subtractive hybridization technique used only produces short reads, which may have reduced the chance of successful matches to conserved areas of the open reading frames. Nevertheless, there remains a good possibility for the discovery of novel biosynthetic enzymes from *D. orbita*.

4.2. Biodistribution of the Secondary Metabolites in D. orbita

Knowledge of the anatomical distribution of natural products is essential for understanding the biosynthesis process and optimal methods for extraction. On a basic level, different tissues can be dissected and extracted to determine which produce and/or store the secondary metabolites. This approach was applied to establish the distribution of Tyrian purple pigments and precursor compounds in the male and female reproductive organs of D. orbita [13]. These compounds were found throughout the female pallial gonoduct [13], with significant quantities in the capsule gland, which lies adjacent to the hypobranchial glands, thus providing evidence for maternal investment of these compounds in the egg masses of D. orbita [4,12]. Despite the production of more oxidized compounds in the male prostate gland, relative to the female gonoduct [13], the presence of significant quantities of these brominated compounds in the males suggests that these compounds are not exclusively produced for defense of the egg masses and likely play some role in the adult life history.

Histochemical techniques for proposed biosynthetic constituents can further aid in establishing the primary metabolic origin of natural products and sites of active biosynthesis [14]. Histomorphological properties of biosynthetic tissues may also reveal regulatory mechanisms, modes of transport, storage and secretion, while histological examination can reveal the presence of potential symbionts (see Section 4.3). The hypobranchial glands of D. orbita show remarkable complexity, with seven distinct types of secretory cells located on the epithelial cell surface [15]. At least two cell types appear to be specifically associated with Tyrian purple synthesis. A subepithelial vascular sinus occurs between the hypobranchial gland and gonoduct, surrounding the rectum and rectal gland [15]. However, there appears to be no direct anatomical mechanism for the transfer of precursors to the gonoduct, suggesting that the compounds are independently synthesized in the reproductive organs. This is supported by the presence of bromoperoxidase and aryl sulfatase activity in the female egg capsule gland [14,18].

Histochemical examination of the biosynthetic enzyme activity and precursors in the hypobranchial glands of *D. orbita* by Westley [18] has further revealed that tyrindoxyl sulfate is biosynthesized through the post-translational bromination of dietary-derived tryptophan, within two discrete sites by two distinct modes. Regulated synthesis occurs on the surface of the lateral hypobranchial epithelium, while the subepithelial vascular sinus of the medial hypobranchial gland appears to constitutively synthesize these compounds. Aryl sulfatase is stored in adjacent supportive cells and exocytosis onto the epithelium surface appears to be regulated [18]. The distinct distribution and regulated activity of aryl sulfatase and bromoperoxidase implies *D. orbita* has evolved the capacity to control the release of bioactive indoles and choline esters. This histological evidence provides further support for a naturally selected role of these secondary metabolites in the life history of the mollusc.

More recently, mass spectrometry imaging (MSI) using desorption/Ionization on porous silicon (DIOS) and nanostructured initiator mass spectrometry (NIMS) was applied to examine the biodistribution of secondary metabolites in *D. orbita* tissues [52]. MSI of biological tissues is becoming a popular tool for biodistributional studies of proteins and pharmaceuticals. However, standard Matrix Assisted Laser Desorption/Ionization Mass Spectrometry (MALDI MS) MSI is challenging for secondary metabolites with low molecular weight due to intense matrix signals, interfering with the detection of signals from the less abundant target compounds. Due to the broad range of polarities in the brominated indoles, *D. orbita* hypobranchial gland chemistry proved to be a good model system for "proof of principle" of a new technique involving direct tissue stamping onto porous silicon and NALDI targets [52]. Ongoing research using this technique is providing interesting insights into the distribution of choline esters and changes the secondary metabolite profile over the reproductive season [104]. Mass spectrometry imaging could also be applied to examine the biodistribution of the bioactive compounds in preclinical trials, as previously done using MALDI with pharmaceutical compounds in rodent models [105].

4.3. Microbial Symbionts

Tyrian purple, a uniquely marine metabolite, is the brominated derivative of the blue dye indigo, derived from plants in the genus *Isatis* and a range of bacteria [106,107]. This appears to be an interesting case of convergent evolution, although the potential role of bacteria in the production of Tyrian purple precursors is yet to be ruled out. To date it has been assumed that muricid molluscs themselves are responsible for the biosynthesis of Tyrian purple [4]. However, over the last decade there has been increasing recognition for the key role of microbial symbionts in the biosynthesis of marine natural products [108]. The rectal gland, which is embedded in the hypobranchial gland of *D. orbita*, contains an abundant supply of the tryptophan precursor and also appears to be associated with bromoperoxidase activity [14,18]. Bacteria have been observed within specialized invaginations of the rectal gland in the muricid *Nucella lapillus* [109]. The positive identification of biosynthetic bacterial symbionts involved in Tyrian purple precursor production would present a paradigm shift, providing new options for large scale sustainable production of these bioactive metabolites and valuable pigments.

Preliminary attempts to culture the bacteria from *Dicathais orbita* using standard techniques have isolated only one species from the hypobranchial gland and three from the rectal gland, compared to 35 from nonbiosynthetic tissues [30]. The sole bacterium isolated from both of these biosynthetic organs was positive for indole production, suggesting a possible role in Tyrian purple synthesis, although further chemical analysis of the culture supernatant is required. It is also possible that the diversity of bacteria in these biosynthetic organs has been underestimated due to specific environmental requirements for growth. The high concentration of mercaptans, such as dimethyl disulfide, in the hypobranchial gland is likely to create a reducing environment [13]. Furthermore, the production of Tyrian purple precursors in culture must require sufficient bromine ion availability. Therefore, a range of novel culture conditions may be required to facilitate the growth and secondary metabolism of Muricidae symbionts. Considering that by far the majority of microorganisms can not be easily cultured [110], the application of culture techniques alone may not be sufficient to identify the diversity of microbial symbionts in *D. orbita*. Metagenomic-based approaches have provided evidence of a microbial origin for several metabolites produced by marine invertebrates [108] and have been successfully applied to the identification of indigo producing bacterial strains in soil [107].

Recent histological and genetic studies have also revealed the presence of ciliate protozoans within the hypobranchial glands of *D. orbita* [21,50]. These ciliates are most likely feeding on bacteria on the epithelial surfaces and interstitial spaces. At present, it is unclear whether these ciliates are pathogens, symbionts or just facultative opportunists. The ciliates do not seem to be directly involved in the production of Tyrian purple based on a lack of histological correlation in the location of the ciliates [21], compared to the biosynthetic enzymes and precursor compounds [18]. However, the abundance of the ciliates does increase towards the reproductive season [21], which correlates with an increase in biosynthetic activity and indole precursor storage prior to spawning [4,12,18,84]. This suggests that the brominated indole precursors could be involved in regulating the activity and/or abundance of ciliates in *D. orbita*. The secondary metabolites from *D. orbita* have not yet been tested for anti-protozoan activity, however a number of other indoles are known to possess anti-parasitic activity [96].

4.4. Sustainable Supply

Tyrian purple is the world's most expensive colorant (1 g = 2439.50 EUR) [111], and is currently extracted from *Purpura lapillus* (10,000 adult snails for 1 g) and South American Muricidae considered at risk from over fishing [89]. The bioactive properties of the brominated indole precursors and the potential for nutraceutical development from the bioactive extracts, provides a further incentive for large-scale sustainable supply. Ecological and life history studies on *D. orbita* [24,31,33,37–39,41,112] contribute to our ability to effectively monitor the population size and recruitment potential of this species. In fact *D. orbita* has been used as a model species for estimating population size [113,114] and for monitoring TBT pollution in the Australian marine environment [32,115,116]. However, as top invertebrate predators, Muricidae molluscs are susceptible to population crashes and the persistence of imposex in some populations further increases their susceptibility to over harvest.

Some progress has been made towards the larval culture [41] and sea-based polyculture of *D. orbita* on abalone farms [40]. However, it has not yet been possible to close the life cycle of this species due to the long planktotrophic (feeding) larval stage and lack of known cues for settlement and metamorphosis [41,117]. Nevertheless, progress has been made towards understanding the growth rates and dietary preferences of the juvenile snails [44,118]. Furthermore, Noble *et al.* [112] have established that it is possible to obtain the bioactive indole precursors from a mucus secretion of *D. orbita*, which offers the potential for non-lethal harvest.

Although generally not suitable for nutraceuticals, chemical synthesis of bioactive metabolites is generally the preferred option for pharmaceutical supply [119]. This can be efficiently achieved for 6-bromoisatin [20,80] and the choline esters [16,62]. These well known molecules can not be patented, but nevertheless provide interesting leads for the chemical synthesis of a range of structural analogues [16,72,79,80,103], thus permitting the assessment of structure activity relationships. Some bioactive marine metabolites are too difficult or expensive to chemically synthesize and previous attempts to chemically synthesis the anticancer precursor of Tyrian purple, tyrindoleninone, have been unsuccessful [16,20]. This is partly due to nonspecific bromination favoring the 5 or 7 position on the indole ring, thus generating low yields for 6-bromoindole derivatives. However, a greater problem occurs in relation to the addition of a methane thiol group at position 2, due to uncontrollable rapid oxidation to 6-bromoisatin. Consequently, tyrindoleninone is not optimal for pharmaceutical development, and holds better potential for human health applications if incorporated into nutraceutical extracts.

The identification of biosynthetic bacteria, enzymes and gene clusters involved in Tyrian purple production could have important implications for application in sustainable production of *D. orbita* brominated indole derivatives, as well as the bioengineering of novel compounds through recombinant expression. Identification of bacterial symbionts that can produce tyrindoxyl sulfate would facilitate the large scale sustainable production of bioactive brominated indoles and Tyrian purple, assuming these bacteria can be cultured. Over the last decade, there have been increasingly frequent reports of gene clusters or gene cassettes for the biosynthesis of marine natural products [108]. Identification of the full gene cluster associated with tyrindoxyl sulphate biosynthesis in Muricidae would open up the potential for recombinant expression of the entire pathway in an heterologous host. This could also facilitate the rational engineering of new metabolites using combinations of enzymes from distinct biosynthetic pathways, which is an important goal for future drug development [98].

5. Conclusions

The Australian Muricidae *D. orbita* biosynthesizes a range of biologically active secondary metabolites, which have stimulated extensive biological and chemical investigations since the 1960s. Early research focused on the identification of the precursors to the well known ancient dye Tyrian purple, and revealed an interesting association between these brominated indole precursors and choline esters. The muscle-relaxant and neurotoxic activity of Muricidae choline esters has been well described in the literature and more recent research has focused on the anticancer properties of the brominated indoles. Despite significant research interest, the ecological and physiological role of the Tyrian purple precursors remains uncertain. However, the combination of biologically active compounds present in *D. orbita* provides interesting potential for nutraceutical development. Increasing biological knowledge on the ecology of the snail, as well as the biodistribution and biosynthesis of secondary metabolites in this species will facilitate sustainable supply. These biological and chemical insights on *D. orbita* provide a good basis for future research and position this species as a suitable model system for novel method development and other innovative research in marine natural product chemistry.

Acknowledgments: Support from the Marine Ecology Research Centre, Southern Cross University and School of Biological Sciences, Flinders University is much appreciated. I would like to thank all of the postgraduate research students and collaborators who have contributed to my research program on *D. orbita* over the last 10 years, my original Ph.D. advisors Andy Davis and John Bremner at the University of Wollongong where this research began, as well as Joe Baker for his inspiration and personal insights on *D. orbita*.

References

1. Baker, J.T. Tyrian purple: An ancient dye, a modern problem. *Endeavour* **1974**, *33*, 11–17. [CrossRef]
2. Cooksey, C.J. Tyrian purple: 6,6′-Dibromoindigo and related compounds. *Molecules* **2001**, *6*, 736–769.
3. Freidlander, P. Ueber den farbstoff des antiken purpura aus *Murex brandaris*. *Chem. Ber.* **1909**, *42*, 765–770. [CrossRef]
4. Westley, C.B.; Vine, K.L.; Benkendorff, K. A Proposed Functional Role for Indole Derivatives in Reproduction and Defense of the Muricidae (Neogastropoda: Mollusca). In *Indirubin, the Red Shade of Indigo*; Meijer, L., Guyard, N., Skaltsounis, L., Eisenbrand, G., Eds.; Station Biologique de Roscoff: Roscoff, France, 2006; pp. 31–44.
5. Laffy, P.W.; Benkendorff, K.; Abbott, C.A. Suppressive subtractive hybridization transcriptomics provides a novel insight into the functional role of the hypobranchial gland in a marine mollusc. *Comp. Biochem. Physiol. Part D Genomics Proteomics* **2013**, *8*, 111–122.
6. Baker, J.; Duke, C. Chemistry of the indoleninones. II. Isolation from the hypobranchial glands of marine molluscs of 6-bromo-2,2-dimethylthioindolin-3-one and 6-bromo-2-methylthioindoleninone as alternative precursors to Tyrian purple. *Aust. J. Chem.* **1973**, *26*, 2153–2157.
7. Baker, J.; Duke, C. Isolation of choline and choline ester salts of tyrindoxyl sulphate from the marine molluscs *Dicathais orbita* and *Mancinella keineri*. *Tetrahedron Lett.* **1976**, *15*, 1233–1234. [CrossRef]
8. Baker, J.; Sutherland, M. Pigments of marine animals VIII. Precursors of 6,6′-dibromoindigotin (Tyrian purple) from the mollusc *Dicathais orbita* (Gmelin). *Tetrahedron Lett.* **1968**, *1*, 43–46. [CrossRef]
9. Baker, J.T. Studies on Tyrian Purple and Its Precursors from Australian Molluscs. Ph.D. Thesis, University of Queensland, Brisbane, Australia, 1967.
10. Baker, J.T.; Duke, C.C. Precursors of Tyrian Purple. In *Food-Drugs Sea*; Marine Technology Society: Washington, DC, USA, 1974; pp. 345–354.
11. Baker, J.T.; Duke, C.C. Isolation from the hypobranchial glands of marine molluscs of 6-bromo-2,2-dimethylthioindolin-3-one and 6-bromo-2-methylthioindoleninone as alternative precursors to Tyrian purple. *Tetrahedron Lett.* **1973**, *14*, 2481–2482. [CrossRef]
12. Benkendorff, K.; Bremner, J.B.; Davis, A.R. Tyrian purple precursors in the egg masses of the Australian muricid, *Dicathais orbita*: A possible defensive role. *J. Chem. Ecol.* **2000**, *26*, 1037–1050. [CrossRef]
13. Westley, C.; Benkendorff, K. Sex-specific Tyrian purple genesis: Precursor and pigment distribution in the reproductive system of the marine mollusc, *Dicathais orbita*. *J. Chem. Ecol.* **2008**, *34*, 44–56. [CrossRef]
14. Westley, C.; Benkendorff, K. The distribution of precursors and biosynthetic enzymes required for Tyrian purple genesis in the hypobranchial gland, gonoduct, an egg masses of *Dicathais orbita* (Gmelin, 1791) (Neogastropoda: Muricidae. *Nautilus* **2009**, *123*, 148–153.
15. Westley, C.B.; Lewis, M.C.; Benkendorff, K. Histomorphology of the hypobranchial gland in *Dicathais orbita* (Gmelin, 1791) (Neogastropoda: Muricidae). *J. Moll. Stud.* **2010**, *76*, 186–195. [CrossRef]
16. Duke, C.C. A Study of Precursors to Purple Dyes from Australian Gastropod Molluscs and of Analogous Synthetic Compounds. Ph.D. Thesis, James Cook University, Townsville, Qld, Australia, 1973.
17. Benkendorff, K. Bioactive Molluscan Resources and Their Conservation: Biological and Chemical Studies on the Egg Masses of Marine Molluscs. Ph.D. Thesis, University of Wollongong, Wollongong, Australia, 1999.

18. Westley, C.B. The Distribution, Biosynthetic Origin and Functional Significance of Tyrian Purple Precursors in the Australian Muricid *Dicathais orbita* (Neogastropoda: Muricidae). Ph.D. Thesis, Flinders University, Adelaide, SA, Australia, 2008.
19. Edwards, V. The Effects of Bioactive Compounds from the Marine Mollusc *Dicathais orbita* on Human Reproductive Cells and Human Reproductive Cancer Cells. Ph.D. Thesis, Flinders University, Adelaide, SA, Australia, 2012.
20. Vine, K.L. An Investigation into the Cytotoxic Properties of Isatin-Derived Compounds: Potential Use in Targeted Cancer Therapy. Ph.D. Thesis, University of Wollongong, Wollongong, NSW, Australia, 2007.
21. Laffy, P.W. Evolution, Gene Expression and Enzymatic Production of Tyrian Purple: A Molecular Study of the Australian Muricid *Dicathais orbita* (Neogastropoda: Muricidae). Ph.D. Thesis, Flinders University, Adelaide, SA, Australia, 2012.
22. Wang, R. Effects of Marine Mollusc Extracts on Human Immune Function. Master's Thesis, Flinders University, Adelaide, SA, Australia, 2009.
23. Vine, K.L. Cytotoxicity of Molluscan Extracts and Natural Products. Biotechnology Honours Thesis, University of Wollongong, Wollongong, NSW, Australia, 2002.
24. Noble, W.J. Survey Methodologies and the Distribution and Abundance of *Dicathais orbita* in South Australia: Population Characteristics and Appropriateness of Techniques. Honours Thesis, Flinders University, Adelaide, SA, Australia, 2004.
25. Laffy, P.W. Genes Expressed in the Hypobranchial Gland of *Dicathais orbita*. Honours Thesis, Flinders University, Adelaide, SA, Australia, 2004.
26. Cocks, R.R. *In Vitro* Bioactivity of Extracts from the Mucus of *Dicathais orbita* against the MCF-7 Breast Cancer Cell Line. Honours Thesis, Flinders University, Adelaide, SA, Australia, 2008.
27. Bogdanovic, A. Isolation of Bioactive Compounds from the Egg Masses of *Dicathais orbita*. Honours Thesis, Flinders University, Adelaide, SA, Australia, 2007.
28. Lim, S.H. Microbial Fouling and Antifouling Properties of Molluscan Egg Masses. Honours Thesis, Flinders University, Adelaide, SA, Australia, 2006.
29. Woodcock, S.H. Dietary Preferences and the Impact of Diet on the Growth and Proximate Composition of the Marine Whelk *Dicathais orbita*. Honours Thesis, Flinders University, Adelaide, SA, Australia, 2007.
30. Roberts, B. Bacterial Communities Associated with the Marine Snail *Dicathais orbita*. Honours Thesis, Flinders University, Adelaide, SA, Australia, 2009.
31. Phillips, B. The Biology of the Whelk *Dicathais* in Western Australia. Ph.D. Thesis, University of Western Australia, Perth, Australia, 1968.
32. Gibson, C.P. The Current Status of Imposex in the Intertidal Gastropod, *Thais orbita* Gmelin (Muricidae), along the New South Wales Coast, Australia. Ph.D. Thesis, Australian Catholic University, Sydney, Australia, 1999.
33. Fairweather, P.G. Interactions between Predators and Prey, and the Structure of Rocky Intertidal Communities. Ph.D. Thesis, University of Sydney, Sydney, Australia, 1985.
34. Przeslawski, R. The Effects of UV Radiation on the Egg Masses of Intertidal Molluscs. Ph.D. Thesis, University of Wollongong, Wollongong, NSW, Australia, 2005.
35. Brown, E. Effects of Human Access on the Size Distribution and Abundance of Intertidal Molluscs along the Fleurieu Peninsula. Honours Thesis, Flinders University, Adelaide, NSW, Australia, 2009.
36. Rittschof, D.; McClellan-Green, P. Molluscs as multidisciplinary models in environment toxicology. *Mar. Poll. Bull.* **2005**, *50*, 369–373. [CrossRef]
37. Phillips, B.F.; Campbell, N.A.; Phillips, B. Mortality and longevity in the whelk *Dicathais orbita* (Gmelin). *Mar. Freshw. Res.* **1974**, *25*, 25–33. [CrossRef]
38. Phillips, B.F.; Campbell, N.A.; Wilson, B.R. A multivariate study of geographic variation in the whelk *Dicathais*. *J. Exp. Mar. Biol. Ecol.* **1973**, *11*, 27–69. [CrossRef]
39. Fairweather, P. Movements of intertidal whelks (*Morula marginalba* and *Thais orbita*) in relation to availability of prey and shelter. *Mar. Biol.* **1988**, *100*, 63–68.
40. Benkendorff, K. Aquaculture and the Production of Pharmaceuticals and Nutraceuticals. In *New Technologies in Aquaculture: Improving Production Efficiency, Quality and Environmental Management*; Burnell, G., Allen, G., Eds.; Woodhead Publishing: Cambridge, UK, 2009; pp. 866–891.

41. Phillips, B.F. The population of the whelk *Dicathais aegrota* in Western Australia. *Mar. Freshw. Res.* **1969**, *20*, 225–266.
42. Westley, C.B.; Lewis, M.C.; Benkendorff, K. Histomorphology of the female pallial gonoduct in *Dicathais orbita* (Neogastropoda, Muricidae): Sperm passage, fertilization, and sperm storage potential. *Invert. Biol.* **2010**, *129*, 138–150.
43. Westley, C.B.; Benkendorff, K. Histochemical correlations between egg capsule laminae and the female gonoduct reveal the process of capsule formation in the Muricidae (Neogastropoda: Mollusca). *Invert. Reprod. Dev.* **2008**, *52*, 81–92. [CrossRef]
44. Woodcock, S.H.; Benkendorff, K. The impact of diet on the growth and proximate composition of juvenile whelks, *Dicathais orbita* (Gastropoda: Mollusca). *Aquaculture* **2008**, *276*, 162–170. [CrossRef]
45. Kool, S.P. Phylogenetic analysis of the Rapaninae (Neogastropoda: Muricidae). *Malacologia* **1993**, *35*, 155–259.
46. Barco, A.; Claremont, M.; Reid, D.G.; Houart, R.; Bouchet, P.; Williams, S.T.; Cruaud, C.; Couloux, A.; Oliverio, M. A molecular phylogenetic framework for the Muricidae, a diverse family of carnivorous gastropods. *Mol. Phylogenet. Evol.* **2010**, *56*, 1025–1039. [CrossRef]
47. Colgan, D.; Ponder, W.; Beacham, E.; Macaranas, J. Gastropod phylogeny based on six segments from four genes representing coding or non-coding and mitochondrial or nuclear DNA. *Moll. Res.* **2003**, *23*, 123–148.
48. Colgan, D.J.; Ponder, W.F.; Beacham, E.; Macaranas, J. Molecular phylogenetics of Caenogastropoda (Gastropoda: Mollusca). *Mol. Phylogenet. Evol.* **2007**, *42*, 717–737. [CrossRef]
49. Colgan, D.J.; Ponder, W.F.; Eggler, P.E. Gastropod evolutionary rates and phylogenetic relationships assessed using partial 28S rDNA and histone H3 sequences. *Zool. Scripta* **2000**, *29*, 29–63. [CrossRef]
50. Laffy, P.W.; Benkendorff, K.; Abbott, C.A. Trends in molluscan gene sequence similiarity: An observation from genes expressed within the hypobranchial gland of *Dicathais orbita* (Gmelin, 1791) (Neogastropoda: Muricidae). *Nautilus* **2009**, *123*, 154–158.
51. Cardenas, L.; Sanchez, R.; Gomez, D.; Fuenzalida, G.; Gallardo-Escarate, C.; Tanguy, A. Transcriptome analysis in *Concholepas concholepas* (Gastropoda, Muricidae): Mining and characterization of new genomic and molecular markers. *Mar. Genomics* **2011**, *4*, 197–205. [CrossRef]
52. Ronci, M.; Rudd, D.; Guinan, T.; Benkendorff, K.; Voelcker, N.H. Mass spectrometry imaging on porous silicon: Investigating the distribution of bioactives in marine mollusc tissues. *Anal. Chem.* **2012**, *84*, 8996–9001.
53. Cole, W. Letter to the Philosophical Society of Oxford containing observations on the purple fish. *Phil. Trans. R. Soc. Lond.* **1685**, *15*, 1278–1286. [CrossRef]
54. Christophersen, C.; Watjen, F.; Buchardt, O.; Anthoni, U. A revised structure of tyriverdin: The precursor to Tyrian purple. *Tetrahedron Lett.* **1978**, *34*, 2779–2781. [CrossRef]
55. Cooksey, C.J. Marine Indirubins. In *Indirubin, the Red Shade of Indigo*; Meijer, L., Guyard, N., Skaltsounis, L., Eisenbrand, G., Eds.; Progress in Life Series: Roscoff, France, 2006; pp. 23–30.
56. Lipinski, C.A.; Lombardo, F.; Dominy, B.W.; Feeney, P.J. Experimental and computational approaches to estimate solubility and permeability in drug discovery and development settings. *Adv.Drug Del. Rev.* **1997**, *23*, 4–25.
57. Baker, J.T. Some metabolites from Australian marine organisms. *Pure Appl. Chem.* **1976**, *48*, 35–44. [CrossRef]
58. Fouquet, H.; Bielig, H.J. Biological precursors and genesis of Tyrian Purple. *Angew. Chem. Int. Ed.* **1971**, *10*, 816–817. [CrossRef]
59. Benkendorff, K.; Westley, C.B.; Gallardo, C.S. Observations on the production of purple pigments in the egg capsules, hypobranchial and reproductive glands from seven species of Muricidae (Gastropoda: Mollusca). *Invert. Reprod. Dev.* **2004**, *46*, 93–102. [CrossRef]
60. Benkendorff, K.; Bremner, J.; Davis, A. Indole derivatives from the egg masses of muricid molluscs. *Molecules* **2001**, *6*, 70–78. [CrossRef]
61. Benkendorff, K.; Pillai, R.; Bremner, J.B. 2,4,5-Tribromo-1*H*-Imidazole in the egg masses of three muricid molluscs. *Nat. Prod. Res.* **2004**, *18*, 427–431. [CrossRef]
62. Duke, C.C.; Eichholzer, J.V.; Macleod, J.K. The synthesis of the isomeric *N*-methyl derivatives of murexine. *Aust. J. Chem.* **1981**, *34*, 1739–1744. [CrossRef]
63. Duke, C.C.; Eichholzer, J.V.; Macleod, J.K. *N*-Methylmurexine-naturally occuring marine compound. *Tetrahedron Lett.* **1978**, *50*, 5047–5048.

64. Roseghini, M.; Severini, C.; Erspamer, G.F.; Erspamer, V. Choline esters and biogenic amines in the hypobranchial gland of 55 molluscan species of the neogastropod Muricoidea superfamily. *Toxicon* **1996**, *34*, 33–55. [CrossRef]
65. Shiomi, K.; Ishii, M.; Shimakura, K.; Nagashima, Y.; Chino, M. Tigloycholine: A new choline ester toxin from the hypobranchial gland of two species of muricid gastropods (*Thais clavigera* and *Thais bronni*). *Toxicon* **1998**, *36*, 795–798.
66. Benkendorff, K.; Davis, A.; Bremner, J. Rapid screening for antimicrobial agents in the egg masses of marine muricid molluscs. *J. Med. Appl. Malac.* **2000**, *10*, 211–223.
67. Bandaranayake, W.M. Mycosporines: Are they nature's sunscreens? *Nat. Prod. Rep.* **1998**, *15*, 159–171. [CrossRef]
68. Shick, J.M.; Dunlap, W.C. Mycosporine-like amino acids and related gadusols: Biosynthesis, accumulation, and UV-protective functions in aquatic organisms. *Annu. Rev. Physiol.* **2002**, *64*, 223–262. [CrossRef]
69. Przeslawski, R.; Benkendorff, K.; Davis, A. A quantitative survey of mycosporine-like amino acids (MAAS) in intertidal egg masses from temperate rocky shores. *J. Chem. Ecol.* **2005**, *31*, 2417–2438. [CrossRef]
70. Benkendorff, K.; Davis, A.R.; Rogers, C.N.; Bremner, J.B. Free fatty acids and sterols in the benthic spawn of aquatic molluscs, and their associated antimicrobial properties. *J. Exp. Mar. Biol. Ecol.* **2005**, *316*, 29–44. [CrossRef]
71. Edwards, V.; Benkendorff, K.; Young, F. Marine compounds selectively induce apoptosis in female reproductive cancer cells but not in primary-derived human reproductive granulosa cells. *Mar. Drugs* **2012**, *10*, 64–83. [CrossRef]
72. Meijer, L.; Skaltsounis, A.L.; Magiatis, P.; Polychronopoulos, P.; Knockaert, M.; Leost, M.; Ryan, X.Z.P.; Vonica, C.A.; Brivanlou, A.; Dajani, R.; *et al.* GSK-3-Selective inhibitors derived from Tyrian purple indirubins. *Chem. Biol.* **2003**, *10*, 1255–1266. [CrossRef]
73. Erspamer, V.; Glasser, A. The pharmacological actions of murexine (urocanylcholine). *Br. J. Pharmcol. Chemother.* **1957**, *12*, 176–184. [CrossRef]
74. Zeisel, S.H.; da Costa, K.A. Choline: An essential nutrient for public health. *Nutr. Rev.* **2009**, *67*, 615–623. [CrossRef]
75. Cooksey, C. The synthesis and properties of 6-bromoindigo: Indigo blue or Tyrian purple? The effect of physical state on the colours of indigo and bromoindigos. *Dyes Hist. Archaeol.* **2001**, *16–17*, 97–104.
76. Benkendorff, K.; Davis, A.R.; Bremner, J.B. Chemical defense in the egg masses of benthic invertebrates: An assessment of antibacterial activity in 39 mollusks and 4 polychaetes. *J. Invert. Path.* **2001**, *78*, 109–118. [CrossRef]
77. Benkendorff, K.; McIver, C.M.; Abbott, C.A. Bioactivity of the Murex homeopathic remedy and of extracts from an Australian muricid mollusc against human cancer cells. *Evid. Based Complement. Altern. Med.* **2011**, *2011*. [CrossRef]
78. Westley, C.B.; McIver, C.M.; Abbott, C.A.; Le Leu, R.K.; Benkendorff, K. Enhanced acute apoptotic response to azoxymethane-induced DNA damage in the rodent colonic epithelium by Tyrian purple precursors A potential colorectal cancer chemopreventative. *Cancer Biol. Ther.* **2010**, *9*, 371–379.
79. Magiatis, P.; Skaltsounis, A.L. From *Hexaplex trunculus* to New Kinase Inhibitory Indirubins. In *In Indirubin, the Red Shade of Indigo*; Meijer, L., Guyard, N., Skaltsounis, A.-L., Eisenbrand, G., Eds.; Life in Progress Editions: Roscoff, France, 2006; pp. 147–156.
80. Vine, K.L.; Locke, J.M.; Ranson, M.; Benkendorff, K.; Pyne, S.G.; Bremner, J.B. *In vitro* cytotoxicity evaluation of some substituted isatin derivatives. *Bioorg. Med. Chem.* **2007**, *15*, 931–938. [CrossRef]
81. Esmaeelian, B. *In-Vitro* and *In-Vivo* Testing of Purified Muricid Mollusc Extract on Colorectal Cancer. Ph.D. Thesis, Flinders University, Adelaide, SA, Australia, 2013.
82. Keyl, M.J.; Whittaker, P. Some pharmacological properties of murexine (urocanoylcholine). *Br. J. Pharmcol.* **1958**, *13*, 103–106.
83. Quilliam, J.P. The mechanism of action of murexine on neuromescular transmission in the frog. *Br. J. Pharmcol.* **1957**, *12*, 338–392.
84. Benkendorff, K. Molluscan Resources: The Past Present and Future Value of Molluscs. In *The Other 99%. The Conservation and Biodiversity of Invertebrates*; Ponder, W., Lunney, D., Eds.; Mosman: Sydney, Australia, 1999; p. 454.

85. Lim, N.S.H.; Everuss, K.J.; Goodman, A.E.; Benkendorff, K. Comparison of surface microfouling and bacterial attachment on the egg capsules of two molluscan species representing Cephalopoda and Neogastropoda. *Aquat. Microb. Ecol.* **2007**, *47*, 275–287. [CrossRef]
86. Przeslawski, R.; Benkendorff, K. The role of surface fouling in the development of encapsulated gastropod embryos. *J. Moll. Stud.* **2005**, *71*, 75–83. [CrossRef]
87. Westley, C.B.; Benkendorff, K.; McIver, C.; Leu, R.K.; Abbott, C.A. Gastrointestinal and hepatotoxicity assessment of an anticancer extract from muricid molluscs. *Evid. Based Complement. Altern. Med.* **2013**, in press.
88. Barnes, D.K.A.; Corrie, A.; Whittington, M.; Carvalho, M.A.; Gell, F. Coastal shellfish resource use in the Quirimba Archipelago, Mozambique. *J. Shellfish Res.* **1998**, *17*, 51–58.
89. Leiva, G.E.; Castilla, J.C. A review of the world marine gastropod fishery: Evolution of catches, management and the Chilean experience. *Rev. Fish Biol. Fish.* **2001**, *11*, 283–300. [CrossRef]
90. Vasconcelos, P.; Carvalho, S.; Castro, M.; Gaspar, M. The artisanal fishery for muricid gastropods (banded murex and purple dye murex) in the Ria Formosa lagoon (Algrave coast, Southern Portugal). *Sci. Mar.* **2008**, *72*, 287–298.
91. Jennings, S.; Kaiser, M.; Reynolds, J. *Marine Fisheries Ecology*; Blackwell Science: Oxford, UK, 2001; p. 11.
92. Benkendorff, K. Molluscan biological and chemical diversity: Secondary metabolites and medicinal resources produced by marine molluscs. *Biol. Rev.* **2010**, *85*, 757–775.
93. Debat, J. Promotion of Analgesic and Sedative Action with 5-Bromoistain. U.S. Patent 3,659,011, 1972.
94. Ryan, W.L. Immunization of animals using choline esters as an immunological adjuvant. U.S. Patent 4,171,353, 1979.
95. O'Connor, K.; Hartmans, E.; Hartmans, S. Indigo formation by aromatic hydrocarbon-degrading bacteria. *Biotechnol. Lett.* **1998**, *20*, 219–223.
96. Gul, W.; Hamann, M.T. Indole alkaloid marine natural products: An established source of cancer drug leas with considerable promise for the control of parasitic, neurological and other diseases. *Life Sci.* **2005**, *78*, 442–453. [CrossRef]
97. Wagner, C.; El Omari, M.; Koenig, G.M. Biohalogenation: Nature's way to synthesize halogenated metabolites. *J. Nat. Prod.* **2009**, *72*, 540–553.
98. Neumann, C.S.; Fujimori, D.G.; Walsh, C.T. Halogenation strategies in natural product biosynthesis. *Chem. Biol.* **2008**, *15*, 99–109. [CrossRef]
99. Jannun, R.; Coe, E.L. Bromoperoxidase from the marine snail, *Murex trunculus*. *Comp. Biochem. Physiol. B Biochem. Mol. Biol.* **1987**, *88*, 917–922.
100. Jannun, R.; Nuwayhid, N.; Coe, E. Biological bromination-bromoperoxidase activity in the murex sea-snail. *Fed. Proc.* **1981**, *40*, 1774.
101. Winter, J.M.; Moore, B.S. Exploring the chemistry and biology of vanadium-dependent haloperoxidases. *J. Biol. Chem.* **2009**, *284*, 18577–18581. [CrossRef]
102. Butler, A.; Carter-Franklin, J.N. The role of vanadium bromoperoxidase in the biosynthesis of halogenated marine natural products. *Nat. Prod. Rep.* **2004**, *21*, 180–188. [CrossRef]
103. Vine, K.L.; Matesic, L.; Locke, J.M.; Ranson, M.; Skropeta, D. Cytotoxic and anticancer activities of isatin and its derivatives: A comprehensive review from 2000–2008. *Anticancer Agents Med. Chem.* **2009**, *9*, 397–414.
104. Rudd, D. Marine Natural Products of *Dicathais orbita*: Developing a Potential Nutraceutical and Understanding the Ecological Significance of Active Compounds within This Species. Flinders University: Adealide, SA, Australia, Unpublished work. 2013.
105. Hsieh, Y.; Li, F.; Korfmacher, W. Mapping pharmaceuticals in rat brain sections using MALDI imaging mass spectrometry. *Methods Mol. Biol.* **2010**, *656*, 147–158. [CrossRef]
106. Balfour-Paul, J. *Indigo*; Fitzroy Dearborn: Chicargo, IL, USA, 2000.
107. Lim, H.K.; Chung, E.J.; Kim, J.C.; Choi, G.J.; Jang, K.S.; Chung, Y.R.; Cho, K.Y.; Lee, S.W. Characterization of a forest soil metagenome clone that confers indirubin and indigo production on *Escherichia coli*. *Appl. Environ. Microb.* **2005**, *71*, 7768–7777. [CrossRef]
108. Lane, A.L.; Moore, B.S. A sea of biosynthesis: Marine natural products meet the molecular age. *Nat. Prod. Rep.* **2011**, *28*, 411–428. [CrossRef]

109. Andrews, E.B. The fine structure and function of the anal gland of the muricid, *Nucella lapillus* (Neogastropoda) and a comparison with that of the trochid *Gibbula cineraria*. *J. Moll. Stud.* **1992**, *58*, 297–313. [CrossRef]
110. Rappe, M.S.; Giovannoni, S.J. The uncultured microbial majority. *Ann. Rev. Microb.* **2003**, *57*, 369–394. [CrossRef]
111. Kremer-Pigmente. Tyrian Purple. Available online: http://www.kremer-pigmente.com/en/pigments/tyrian-purple-36010.html (accessed on 24 January 2012).
112. Noble, W.J.; Cocks, R.R.; Harris, J.O.; Benkendorff, K. Application of anaesthetics for sex identification and bioactive compound recovery from wild *Dicathais orbita*. *J. Exp. Mar. Biol. Ecol.* **2009**, *380*, 53–60. [CrossRef]
113. Phillips, B.F.; Campbell, N.A. A new method of fitting the von Bertalanffy growth curve using data on the whelk *Dicathais*. *Growth* **1968**, *32*, 317–329.
114. Phillips, B.F.; Campbell, N.A. Comparison of methods of estimating population size using data on the whelk *Dicathais aegrota* (Reeve). *J. Anim. Ecol.* **1970**, *39*, 753–759. [CrossRef]
115. Gibson, C.P.; Wilson, S.P. Imposex still evident in eastern Australia 10 years after tributyltin restrictions. *Mar. Environ. Res.* **2003**, *55*, 101–112. [CrossRef]
116. Rees, C.M.; Brady, B.A.; Fabris, G.J. Incidence of imposex in *Thais orbita* from Port Phillip Bay (Victoria, Australia), following 10 years of regulation on use of TBT. *Mar. Poll. Bull.* **2001**, *42*, 873–878. [CrossRef]
117. Noble, W.J. Life History Assessment and Larval Culture of *Dicathais orbita*. Flinders University: Adelaide, SA, Australia, Unpublished work. 2013.
118. Morton, B. Competitive grazers and the predatory whelk (Gastropoda: Muricidae) structure a mussel bed on a southwest Australian shore. *J. Moll. Stud.* **1999**, *65*, 435–452. [CrossRef]
119. Sipkema, D.; Osinga, R.; Schatton, W.; Mendola, D.; Tramper, J.; Wijffels, R. Large-scale production of pharmaceuticals by marine sponges: Sea, cell, or synthesis. *Biotechnol. Bioeng.* **2005**, *90*, 201–222.

marine drugs

MDPI

Review

Computational Studies of Marine Toxins Targeting Ion Channels

M. Harunur Rashid, Somayeh Mahdavi and Serdar Kuyucak *

School of Physics, University of Sydney, New South Wales 2006, Australia;
harun@physics.usyd.edu.au (M.H.R.); mahdavi@physics.usyd.edu.au (S.M.)
* Author to whom correspondence should be addressed; serdar@physics.usyd.edu.au; Tel.: +61-2-9036-5306; Fax: +61-2-9036-7158.

Received: 19 December 2012; in revised form: 30 January 2013; Accepted: 7 February 2013;
Published: 13 March 2013

Abstract: Toxins from marine animals offer novel drug leads for treatment of diseases involving ion channels. Computational methods could be very helpful in this endeavour in several ways, e.g., (i) constructing accurate models of the channel-toxin complexes using docking and molecular dynamics (MD) simulations; (ii) determining the binding free energies of toxins from umbrella sampling MD simulations; (iii) predicting the effect of mutations from free energy MD simulations. Using these methods, one can design new analogs of toxins with improved affinity and selectivity properties. Here we present a review of the computational methods and discuss their applications to marine toxins targeting potassium and sodium channels. Detailed examples from the potassium channel toxins—ShK from sea anemone and κ-conotoxin PVIIA—are provided to demonstrate capabilities of the computational methods to give accurate descriptions of the channel-toxin complexes and the energetics of their binding. An example is also given from sodium channel toxins (μ-conotoxin GIIIA) to illustrate the differences between the toxin binding modes in potassium and sodium channels.

Keywords: conotoxins; ShK toxin; ion channels; docking; molecular dynamics; potential of mean force; free energy perturbation

1. Introduction

Voltage-gated ion channels play key roles in electrical signalling in cells. They function much like transistors—A change in the membrane potential opens the channel gate and allows passive diffusion of a selected type of ions such as Na^+,K^+, or Ca^{2+} across the cell membrane [1]. Dysfunction of ion channels due to mutations in the channel protein or environmental effects are associated with numerous diseases [2]. Thus ion channels are important targets for therapeutic drugs, and there is an ongoing interest in the pharmaceutical industry to find channel blockers with high affinity and specificity. Many toxins from marine animals bind to specific ion channels with high affinity [3,4], and therefore provide natural leads for drug development [5–10].

Once a toxin is identified as a potential drug lead for a target ion channel, more work needs to be done to improve its affinity and selectivity for the target. This is essential to reduce the dosage and avoid side effects that may arise from binding of the drug to unintended proteins. This may be achieved in the lab by creating analogs of the toxin through mutations of selected residues, and testing their affinity for various proteins. Such a trial and error approach could be very time consuming and success is not guaranteed. Provided the structures of the target proteins are available—either from X-ray diffraction or via homology modelling—one can alternatively use computational methods to construct accurate models for the channel-toxin complexes and predict the effect of the mutations in silico. Advances in crystallization of membrane proteins and computer hardware/software in the last fifteen years have made such a computational approach to drug design a distinct possibility.

Availability of a crystal structure of an ion channel is essential for computational studies of toxin binding. Channel models constructed in the absence of a crystal structure are not reliable enough to use in atomistic simulations. The first crystal structure of a bacterial potassium channel (KcsA) was determined in 1998 [11], followed by many others [12]. Of particular importance for toxin binding studies was the solution of the mammalian voltage-gated potassium channel Kv1.2 [13], which has enabled construction of homology models for other Kv1 channels. Sodium channels were relatively harder to crystallize. The first crystal structure for a bacterial voltage-gated sodium channel appeared only recently [14], and a mammalian one is yet to be solved. Unlike potassium channels where the pore domains of bacterial and mammalian channels are very similar, there are substantial differences between the two classes in sodium channels. Thus constructing homology models of the mammalian Nav1 channels from the bacterial crystal structure will be a more challenging task. As yet, there are no crystal structures for the calcium channels and the ligand-gated ion channels, which explains the current focus of the computational studies on the potassium and sodium channels.

The most important progress in computer hardware was the introduction of the cluster architecture and parallel computing, which brought supercomputing power to masses. This was an essential breakthrough because an accurate description of structure and dynamics of a complex system requires an atomic-level treatment via molecular dynamics (MD) simulations and sufficient sampling of the simulation system. Routine simulation of a protein system consisting of $\sim 10^5$ atoms in the microsecond range would not have been feasible without the high-performance computing power afforded by the clusters. On the software front, MD programs and their associated force fields such as AMBER [15], CHARMM [16], and GROMACS [17] have been continuously improved since their inception. Used in combination with a docking program, MD simulations have the ability to produce accurate models of protein-ligand complexes [18]. Similarly, one can perform free energy simulations to predict the absolute free energy of binding for a given complex, and predict the change in the binding free energy due to a mutation in the complex near chemical accuracy [19–22].

Here we present a review of the computational methods used in construction of channel-toxin complexes, and calculation of absolute and relative binding free energies in such complexes. Because application of these methods to protein-peptide complexes are relatively new, we provide detailed examples from the potassium channel toxins ShK and κ-conotoxin PVIIA. Computational investigation of sodium channel toxins is just starting. Nevertheless, we give an example from μ-conotoxin GIIIA to illustrate how the binding modes in sodium channels differ from those in potassium channels.

2. Computational Methods

There are only a few crystal structures for complexes of membrane proteins. Thus the first step in a computational study of toxin binding to ion channels is the construction of complex structures. Here accuracy of the model structure is of utmost importance because without an accurate complex model, free energy calculations in the next step have no chance of succeeding. Accordingly, we first discuss the computational methods used in structure prediction followed by the free energy methods.

2.1. Complex Structure Prediction from Docking and MD Simulations

In order to find the structure of a channel-toxin complex, one first needs the individual structures of the channel and the toxin. Those of toxins can be determined using NMR in a straightforward manner, and many toxin structures are available from the protein data bank. Structures of channel proteins are determined from X-ray crystallography, and because it is much harder to crystallize membrane proteins, not many channel structures are available. Hence, one has to rely on homology modeling in most cases. The situation is relatively better in potassium channels where several crystal structures exist [12], including the mammalian voltage-gated potassium channel Kv1.2 [13]. Thus one can construct homology models of other Kv1 channels relatively easily, although it is still very important to validate such model channels using available functional data. In sodium channels, the crystal structure of a bacterial channel was determined recently [14], which has opened the way for homology modelling of the mammalian Nav1 channels. Due to substantial differences between the bacterial and mammalian sodium channels, proper validation of the homology models is even more important in this case.

Two main methods for prediction of protein-ligand complexes are docking and MD simulations. Docking programs allow fast screening of many ligands for a given target [23,24], but their accuracy is limited [25]. Conversely, MD simulations provide accurate representation of the protein-ligand interactions but they are too slow to predict the complex structure from scratch. Combination of the two methods, where the initial binding poses predicted by a docking method are refined in subsequent MD simulations, offers the most practical approach for finding complex structures. Initial applications of this approach to small ligands (< 50 atoms) using common docking programs such as AUTODOCK [26] and ZDOCK [27] produced promising results [18,28–30]. Its feasibility for larger and more flexible peptide ligands was first shown for the KcsA potassium channel-charybdotoxin complex [31,32]. The structure of this complex was determined from NMR experiments [33], so it could be used for testing the accuracy of the docking plus MD approach and the effectiveness of the docking programs [32]. Using a more sophisticated docking program such as HADDOCK [34,35], which allowed flexibility and ensemble docking, was found to give superior results compared with rigid docking programs [28,32].

Docking programs rank the complex poses according to their energy score. Inspection of the top 10 or 20 poses is usually sufficient to make a decision on an initial pose. A systematic study of potassium channel-toxin complexes using HADDOCK has shown that a consensus complex is obtained in most cases [32]. We assume this to be the case in the following, but if more than one pose is found from docking, each pose needs to be refined with MD. After an initial configuration for the complex structure is chosen from docking, one needs to prepare the simulation system for refinement with MD. There are well-established protocols for this purpose [36,37], which can be used for the complex model as well. Typically, the complex model is embedded in a lipid bilayer and solvated with a salt solution using the VMD program [38]. The resulting system is gradually relaxed in MD simulations until it reaches equilibrium. Care needs to be exercised to ensure that all the disulfide and hydrogen bonds in the complex structure are preserved during relaxation. Once the system is well equilibrated in MD simulations, a production run is performed for analysis of the binding mode. Snapshots of the complex system can be used to get a visual picture of the binding mode. A more quantitative description can be obtained by calculating the average pair distances for the strongly interacting residues. Charge interactions, where the N–O distance between the charged residues is less than 3 Å, and hydrophobic interactions involving the benzyl groups provide the strongest couplings (> 2 kcal/mol). Hydrogen bonds and charge interactions at larger distances are of intermediate strength (1–2 kcal/mol). Where available, comparison of the alanine scanning mutagenesis data with the predictions of the complex model provides the best validation for the proposed model. If no mutation data are available, one has to rely on binding free energies, which is discussed in the next section.

There are several MD programs that one can use for refinement of the complex. In the examples discussed here, the NAMD code [39] is used with the CHARMM force field [16] including the CMAP correction for the dihedral terms [40]. The NpT ensemble is the most suitable one for MD simulations of biomolecules and has been adapted in most MD studies. The temperature and pressure can be maintained at the standard values of 300 K and 1 atm using temperature and pressure coupling. Employment of the periodic boundary conditions avoids artefacts arising from using small boundary boxes and also facilitates computation of the long-range electrostatic interactions. Neglecting the long-range electrostatic interactions using cut-off distances causes errors and is not recommended. The current practice is to include them using the particle-mesh Ewald algorithm. The short-range Lennard-Jones interactions can be switched off within a distance of 10–13.5 Å without causing errors. A typical time step used in the MD simulations is 2 fs. Using longer time steps results in accumulation of systematic errors while shorter ones require more computing time and are not used unless extreme accuracy is desired. For details of the basic formalism of MD simulations, we refer to the monographs [41–43]. A recent review of MD simulations of membrane proteins can be found in [44].

2.2. Free Energy Calculations

Binding constants of toxins are routinely measured and readily available for most channel-toxin complexes. Thus, in the absence of mutation data, they provide the only means for validating a complex model. This, in turn, requires an accurate calculation of the binding constant. There are two classes of methods that can be used for this purpose: (i) path independent alchemical perturbation methods, where the ligand is simultaneously destroyed in the binding pocket while created in bulk; and (ii) path dependent potential of mean force (PMF) methods, where the ligand is physically pulled from the binding pocket to bulk [19,20]. Here the PMF gives the continuous free energy profile of the toxin along the chosen reaction coordinate. The first method is computationally cheaper but its application to peptide toxins—which are flexible and have many charged residues—suffers from sampling problems [45]. Thus until the problems in applying the perturbation method to charged-flexible ligands are resolved, the PMF approach will remain the method of choice.

Formally, the binding constant is determined from the 3-D integral of the PMF of the ligand, W (r)

$$K_{eq} = \int_{site} e^{-W(\mathbf{r})/k_B T} \, d^3 r \tag{1}$$

where it is assumed that $W = 0$ in bulk. Because computation of a 3-D PMF is not feasible, one invokes a 1-D approximation and determines the PMF along the reaction coordinate, which is the channel axis for a channel-toxin complex. Taking the channel axis along the z axis, the binding constant is given by

$$K_{eq} = \pi R^2 \int_{z_1}^{z_2} e^{-W(z)/k_B T} \, dz \tag{2}$$

where z_1 and z_2 refer to the toxin's center of mass (COM) coordinates at the binding site and in the bulk, respectively. The factor πR^2 measures the average cross-sectional area of the binding pocket as explored by the COM of the toxin, and the radius R is determined from the transverse fluctuations of the COM of the toxin in the binding pocket. The accuracy of this approximation has been checked for ions by independent free energy perturbation calculations [46]. Because toxins are much heavier, their transverse fluctuations along the z axis are further suppressed compared with ions, so the 1-D approximation should work even better for toxins. The absolute binding free energy is determined from the binding constant using

$$G_b = -k_B T \ln(K_{eq} C_0) \tag{3}$$

where C_0 is the standard concentration of 1 mol/liter (*i.e.*, $1/C_0 = 1661$ Å^3).

The most common method used in PMF calculations is the umbrella sampling MD simulations, where one introduces harmonic potentials to enhance sampling of the ligand at high-energy points [47]. For convenience, umbrella potentials are introduced at regular intervals (e.g., 0.5 Å) along the reaction coordinate. To generate the simulation windows, a harmonic force with k in the range of 20–40 kcal/mol/ Å^2 is applied to the COM of the toxin backbone, which is pulled at a constant speed of 5 Å/ns over 0.5 Å. After each pulling step, the toxin is equilibrated at the window position by applying the same harmonic restraint for 200 ps to relax the effect of steering on the environment. Initially windows are generated for up to 15 Å starting from the binding pocket, which are extended further if necessary (*i.e.*, until the PMF becomes flat). If insufficient overlap occurs between the adjoining windows (typically less than 5%) due to a local potential barrier, an extra window is included in the middle of the two windows. The COM coordinates of the toxin, measured with respect to the COM of the channel, are collected during the umbrella sampling MD simulations. The PMF is obtained using the weighted histogram analysis method [48], which unbiases the COM coordinates in each window and combines them in an optimal way. Convergence of the PMF is the sole criterion on how long one should run each window, which can be studied using block data analysis. Typically PMF obtained from individual blocks of data first monotonically decreases and then fluctuates around a base line. In the first phase, the system is still equilibrating and the data should be discarded. Fluctuations in the second phase indicate that equilibration has been reached, so the final PMF should be constructed using the production data from this part.

An alternative method for constructing the PMF of a ligand is to use Jarzynski's equation [49] in steered MD simulations [50]. Due to its simplicity, this method has become quite popular in recent years. However, detailed comparisons with the umbrella sampling method indicate that its application to biomolecules suffers from sampling problems and the convergence of PMFs is too slow to be useful in practice [51,52].

The PMF method was first applied to the KcsA potassium channel-charybdotoxin complex, where the structure was known, hence providing an important test case [31]. In this study, a large discrepancy was found in the calculated absolute binding free energy, which was caused by the distortion of the toxin during umbrella sampling simulations. In a follow-up study, conformational restraints were used to prevent the deformation of the toxin, which enabled calculation of the absolute binding free energy within chemical accuracy of 1 kcal/mol [53]. Since then, the PMF method has been used in several computational studies of toxin binding to ion channels [54–61]. As long as a validated complex structure was employed in the PMF calculations, the absolute binding free energy was obtained within chemical accuracy in all cases.

Improving the affinity and selectivity of a drug lead via mutations poses a less taxing computational problem, as one is interested in the change in the binding free energy due to a mutation. Provided the binding mode is not altered by the mutation, this is most efficiently calculated using the alchemical transformation methods such as free energy perturbation (FEP) and thermodynamic integration (TI) [62]. In both methods, one introduces a hybrid Hamiltonian, $H(\lambda) = (1 - \lambda)H_0 + \lambda H_1$, where H_0 represents the Hamiltonian in the initial state (wild type ligand) and H_1 in the final state (mutant ligand). The alchemical transformation is performed by changing the parameter λ from 0 to 1 in small steps, which ensures that the change in the free energy in each step is small enough to enable sufficient sampling of the system in a reasonable time frame. In the FEP method, the interval [0,1] is divided into n subintervals with $\{\lambda i, i = 1, n - 1\}$, and for each subinterval the free energy difference is calculated from the ensemble average

$$\Delta G_i = -kT \ln\langle \exp[-(H(\lambda_{i+1}) - H(\lambda_i))/k_B T] \rangle_{\lambda_i} \tag{4}$$

The free energy difference between the initial and final states is obtained from the sum, $\Delta G = \Sigma_i \Delta G_i$. The number of subintervals (windows) is chosen such that the free energy change at each step does not exceed 2 kcal/mol, otherwise the method may lose its validity. For mutations of involving charged residues, this requires over hundred windows if uniform subintervals are used. Using exponentially spaced subintervals instead, one could reduce the number of windows substantially.

In the TI method, the ensemble average of the derivative, $\partial H(\lambda)/\partial\lambda$, is obtained at several λ values, and the free energy difference is calculated from the integral,

$$\Delta G = \int_0^1 \left\langle \frac{\partial H(\lambda)}{\partial \lambda} \right\rangle_\lambda d\lambda \tag{5}$$

The TI method is especially advantageous for mutations involving charged residues, because Gaussian quadrature allows evaluation of the integral using a small number of windows, which can be sampled for longer times to check convergence of the results. A seven-point quadrature was found to be adequate in previous applications of the TI method [46,63]. In both methods, it is important to perform the backward calculation to check for hysteresis effects. If the difference between the forward and backward results is much larger than 1 kcal/mol, the calculated free energies are not reliable, most likely due to insufficient sampling of the system.

Mutation of a charged residue to a neutral one is a more challenging problem and requires additional considerations to avoid sampling problems. Firstly, one needs to preserve the net charge in the system during the calculations. This can be achieved by performing the following thermodynamic cycle: While a charged residue on the toxin in the binding site is mutated to a neutral one, the reverse transformation is simultaneously applied to a mutant toxin in bulk. Secondly, the Coulomb and Lennard-Jones (LJ) interactions need to be handled separately, which can be implemented by introducing uncharged residues as intermediate steps. For example, the free energy change due to a Lys to Ala ($K \rightarrow A$) mutation can be expressed as

$$\Delta\Delta G = \Delta\Delta G(K \rightarrow K^0) + \Delta\Delta G(K^0 \rightarrow A^0) + \Delta\Delta G(A^0 \rightarrow A) \tag{6}$$

The first term represents the discharging of the side chain of a Lys residue on the bound toxin while the reverse process is performed on a toxin in bulk with an uncharged Lys side chain. In the second term, the uncharged Lys side chain is transformed to an uncharged Ala side chain while the reverse is performed on the bulk toxin. Finally, the third term corresponds to charging of the Ala side chain in binding site while the one in bulk is discharged. Each of these contributions to the free energy difference can be calculated using the FEP or TI methods.

3. Potassium Channel Toxins

Due to earlier availability of crystal structures, potassium channels have been the main focus in computational investigations of marine toxins targeting ion channels. Homology models of the voltage-gated potassium channels Kv1 can be constructed using the crystal structure of the Kv1.2 channel in a straightforward manner. As shown in Table 1, there is one-to-one correspondence among the pore domain residues, thus the models can be simply constructed using the mutator plugin in the VMD software [38]. The only important point to note in modeling of the Kv1 channels is the residue following the DM signature in the extended region, which corresponds to T449 in Shaker, Y379 in Kv1.1, V381 in Kv1.2, and H404 in Kv1.3. In both Shaker and Kv1.3 the side chain of this residue makes a cross-link with the side chain of the neighboring D residue (*i.e.*, T449–D447 in Shaker and H404–D402 in Kv1.3). There is no such cross-linking in Kv1.1 because the Y379 side chain is too bulky to fit around the filter. If the models of Shaker and Kv1.3 are not properly relaxed in MD simulations, these cross-links could break, resulting in a wrong model of the channel, where the T449/H404 side chains project out of the pore. The protruding T449/H404 side chains interfere with the binding of toxins and prevent their correct docking to Shaker [64] and Kv1.3 channels [54,55].

Table 1. Alignment of the Shaker and rat Kv1 channel sequences depicting the differences in the turret and extended regions.

		Turret	Pore helix	Filter	Extended region	
Shaker	418	EAGSENSFFK	SIPDAFWWAVVTMTTVGYG		DMT PVGVW	454
Kv1.1	348	EAEEAESHFS	SIPDAFWWAVVSMTTVGYG		DMYPV T I G	384
Kv1.2	350	EADERDSQFP	SIPDAFWWAVVSMTTVGYG		DMVPT T I G	386
Kv1.3	373	EADDPSSGFN	SIPDAFWWAVVTMTTVGYG		DMHPV T I G	409

In this section we discuss binding of ShK toxin from sea anemone and κ-conotoxin PVIIA to Kv1 potassium channels in some detail to show that computational methods can provide accurate descriptions of the channel-toxin complexes and the energetics of their binding. These examples are chosen because of the availability of the alanine scanning mutagenesis data, which allow a direct validation of the proposed complex models. NMR structures of ShK [65] and PVIIA [66] are shown in Figure 1.

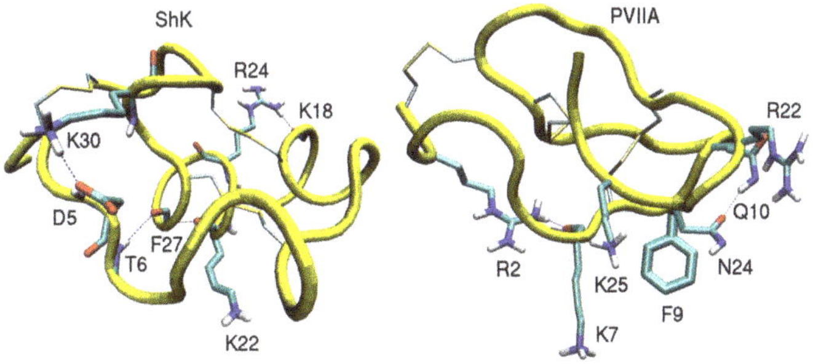

Figure 1. NMR structures of the ShK toxin and κ-conotoxin PVIIA oriented with the pore inserting lysine pointing downward. In ShK, there are three disulfide bonds (C3–C35, C12–C28, and C17–C32), and three other bonds (D5–K30, K18–R24 and T6–F27), which make the structure very stable. In PVIIA, there are three disulfide bonds (C1–C16, C8–C20, and C15–C26), and two other bonds (R2–K7 and Q10–N24).

3.1. ShK Toxin

The Kv1.3 channel is an established target for the treatment of autoimmune diseases, such as multiple sclerosis and rheumatoid arthritis [67,68]. ShK toxin from the sea anemone Stichodactyla helianthus [69,70] binds to the Kv1.3 channel with an $IC5_0$ of 11 pM [71], hence it provides an excellent lead for development of an immunosuppressant drug. However, ShK also binds to other Kv channels with high affinity, in particular Kv1.1 with an $IC5_0$ of 16 pM [71]. Lack of specificity for Kv1.3 prevents the use of ShK as a therapeutic drug. Therefore, there is an intense effort for developing analogs of ShK that have improved selectivity for Kv1.3 over Kv1.1 and other potassium channels [9,10]. Many ShK analogs have been created for this purpose, and some had the required selectivity, e.g., ShK-Dap22 [71], ShK-186 [72], and ShK-192 [73]. However, the use of non-natural amino acids or adducts in these analogs has limited their potential for development as drugs. For example, the phosphorylated Tyr residue in ShK-186 is prone to hydrolysis. Therefore, developing Kv1.3 selective analogs of ShK from natural amino acids is more desirable.

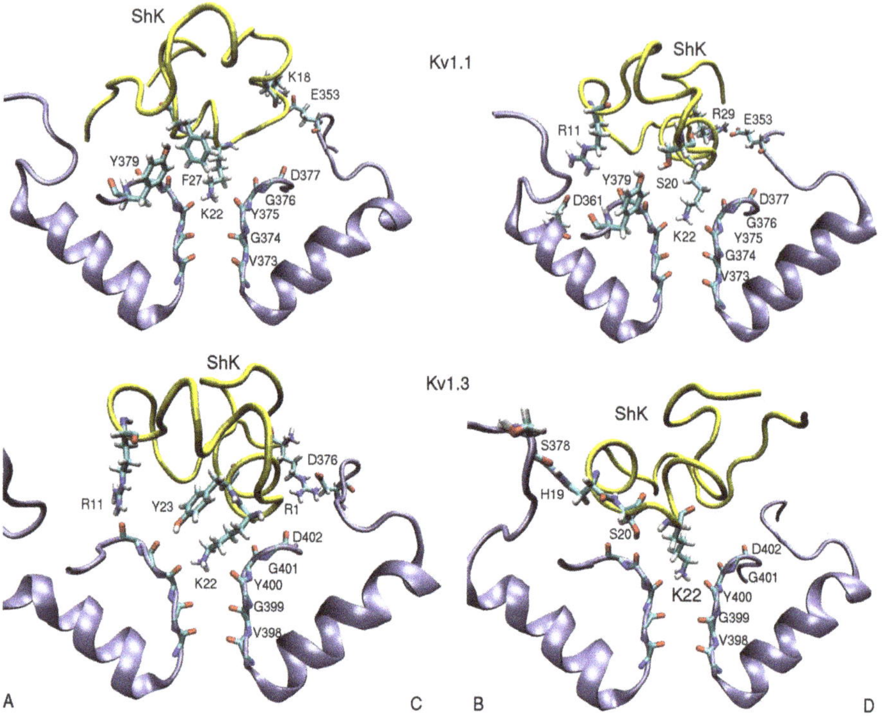

Figure 2. Snapshots of the Kv1.1–ShK and Kv1.3–ShK complexes showing the strongly interacting residues. Only those involved in the binding are indicated explicitly. In order to show all the residues involved in binding, two views of the complex are presented depicting the channel monomers A and C, and B and D separately.

An essential first step in searching for selective analogs using structure-based drug design methods is to construct accurate models of the protein-ligand complexes involved in the selectivity problem. This has been recently achieved for the Kv1.x–ShK complexes using docking and molecular dynamics (MD) simulations [59]. Snapshots of the equilibrated Kv1.1–ShK and Kv1.3–ShK complexes are shown in Figure 2. A more quantitative description of the strongly interacting residues is provided in Table 2, which shows the average atom-atom distances obtained from 5 ns of unrestrained MD simulations for each complex. Comparison of the results for the Kv1.3–ShK complex with the alanine scanning mutagenesis data [74] shows that the complex model accounts for all the strongly interacting residues identified in the experiment. The only exception is the mutation R24A, which is an allosteric effect. R24 is not involved in the binding but its mutation to alanine breaks the R24–K18 bond (see Figure 1), which changes the shape of the ShK mutant and its binding mode. Further evidence for the validity of the complex models are provided by the binding free energies, which are obtained from the integration of the PMFs shown in Figure 3. In all three cases, the PMF calculations of the binding free energies have reproduced the experimental values within chemical accuracy [59].

Table 2. List of the strongly interacting residues in the ShK–Kv1.x complexes. The average atom-atom distances obtained from MD simulations are given in units of Å (standard deviations are not listed as they are less than 0.4 Å). The N–O distances are shown for the charge interactions and the closest C–C distance for the hydrophobic ones. Bare C, N, and O refer to the backbone atoms and the subscripted ones refer to the side chain atoms. The monomer identity is given at the end of the residue number.

ShK–Kv1.1	dist.	ShK–Kv1.2	dist.	ShK–Kv1.3	dist.
				R1(N_1)–D376(O_1)C	4.5
R11(N_2)–D361(O_2)B	5.5	S10(O_H)–D353(O_2)B	2.8	R11(N_2)–D402(O)A	3.5
K18(N_1)–E353(O_2)C	2.7			H19(N)–S378(O)B	3.0
S20(O_H)–Y379(O_H)B	3.0	M21(N)–D379(O)D	3.1	S20(O_H)–G401(O)B	2.7
		M21(C_γ)–V381($C_{\gamma 2}$)D	3.8	M21(C_ε)–V406($C_{\gamma 1}$)B	4.7
K22(N_1)–Y375(O)	2.7	K22(N_1)–Y377(O)	2.7	K22(N_1)–Y400(O)	2.7
				Y23(O_H)–G401(O)A	3.5
F27($C_{\varepsilon 2}$)–Y379($C_{\varepsilon 1}$)A	3.6			F27($C_{\varepsilon 1}$)–H404-C_γ)C	3.6
R29(N_2)–E353(O_2)D	2.5	R29(N_1)–D355(O_1)A	2.7	R29(N_1)–D376(O_1)C	10.2

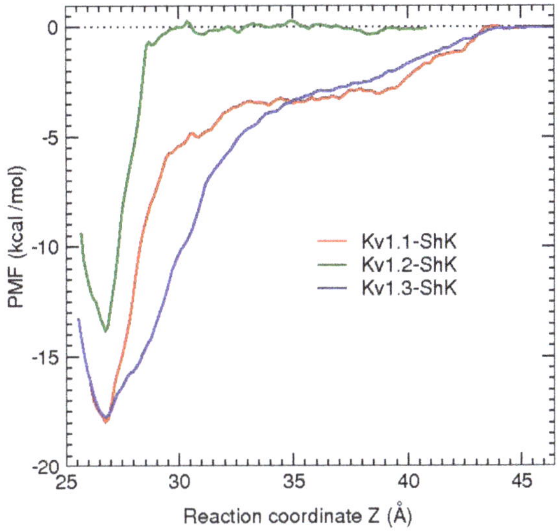

Figure 3. Comparison of the PMFs obtained from the umbrella sampling simulations for the unbinding of ShK from the Kv1.1, Kv1.2, and Kv1.3 channels.

Comparison of the binding modes of the Kv1.1–ShK and Kv1.3–ShK complexes (Figure 2 and Table 2) gives valuable hints for improving the selectivity of ShK for Kv1.3 over Kv1.1. The side chains of K18 and R29 in ShK are strongly coupled to the glutamate side chains in Kv1.1 via ionic bonds but they do not exhibit any interactions with the Kv1.3 residues. Thus mutation of the either residue in ShK to alanine could lead to a substantial selectivity gain for Kv1.3 over Kv1.1. To test this hypothesis, binding of the K18A and R29A mutants of ShK to the Kv1 channels have been studied employing the same protocols used for ShK. The R29A mutation was found to alter the binding mode in both Kv1.1 and Kv1.3, and therefore was not pursued. The K18A mutation did preserve the binding mode in both channels, and hence the effect of the K18A mutation on the selectivity free energy could be calculated using the FEP and TI methods. Because the validity of these methods for charge mutations was not well established, the binding free energies of ShK-K18A were also calculated as a test of FEP and TI. All three methods gave similar results and predicted that the K18A mutation would improve the Kv1.3/Kv1.1 selectivity free energy by about 2 kcal/mol, which was confirmed in subsequent experiments.

An amidated analogue of ShK (ShK-K-amide) has been known to improve the Kv1.3/Kv1.1 selectivity but the mechanism of this selectivity was not clear. A similar computational study performed for ShK-K-amide showed that this mutation had negligible effect on its binding to Kv1.3 but grossly altered its binding mode to Kv1.1 [60]. The binding free energies of ShK-K-amide calculated from the respective PMFs again reproduced the experimental values within chemical accuracy, increasing the confidence in the accuracy of the computational methods.

3.2. κ-conotoxin PVIIA

The drosophila Shaker (Shaker) channel is the first voltage-gated potassium channel to be cloned, and therefore it is often used as a role model in investigation of the structure and function of potassium channels. Similarly, κ-PVIIA is the first conotoxin found to block Shaker [75], and thus it has attracted a great deal of attention. The binding mode of κ-PVIIA to Shaker was studied via mutagenesis experiments [76,77], and it has also been used in many functional studies of Shaker channels [78–81]. Structure and mutagenesis data indicate that κ-PVIIA binds to Shaker via a functional dyad consisting of a pore-inserting lysine (K7) and a hydrophobic residue (F9), similar to the binding mode of other toxin blockers of potassium channels [82,83]. In an earlier computational study of the Shaker-κ-PVIIA complex [64], the functional dyad was reproduced but the other important interactions identified in the mutagenesis experiments [77] were not. As stressed earlier, this was due to incorrect modelling of the pore region of Shaker.

In a more recent study of κ-PVIIA binding to Shaker and Kv1 channels [61], a correct model of Shaker was used and the results obtained from the Shaker-κ-PVIIA complex model were in general agreement with the experiments. Similar protocols as in ShK were employed in creating the complex model. Snapshots of the Shaker-κ-PVIIA complex is shown in Figure 4. The pairs of residues involved in binding and the average distances between the pairs of atoms—obtained from the MD simulations of the complex—are given in Table 3. Comparison of the pairs of residues in Table 3 with the alanine scanning mutagenesis data [77] shows that all strongly interacting residues identified in the experiment have been accounted for in the complex structure. The binding energies of κ-PVIIA to Shaker and Kv1.2 have also been reproduced within chemical accuracy, providing further validation for the complex models.

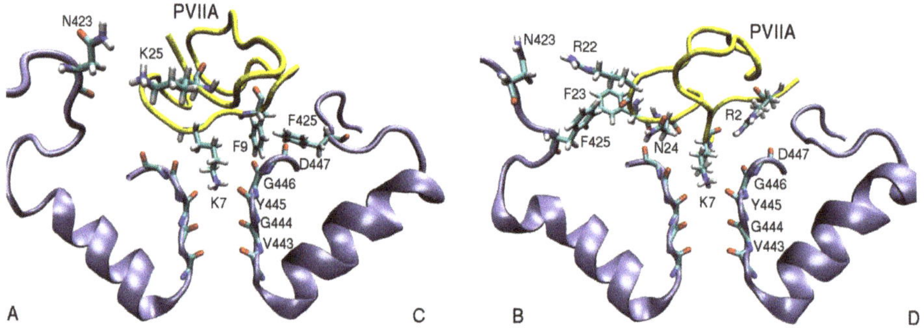

Figure 4. Snapshots of the Shaker-κ-PVIIA complex showing the important residues involved in binding. The monomers A and C and B and D are shown separately for clarity.

Table 3. Similar to Table 2 but for the κ-PVIIA–Kv1 complexes. Benz refers to the COM of the benzyl group.

κ-PVIIA–Shaker	dist.	κ-PVIIA–Kv1.1	dist.	κ-PVIIA–Kv1.2	dist.
R2(N_1)–D447(O)D	3.9	R2(N_2)–D377(O)A	5.0	R2(N_2)–D379(O)D	3.7
Q6(N_1)–D447(O)A	4.7	Q6(N_1)–D377(O)A	5.1	Q6(N_1)–D379(O)A	3.2
K7(N_1)–Y445(O)	2.7	K7(N_1)–Y375(O)	2.8	K7(N_1)–Y377(O)	2.7
F9(C_ζ)–T449($C_{\gamma 2}$)C	4.4	F9($C_{\delta 2}$)–Y379($C_{\epsilon 2}$)C	3.9	F9($C_{\epsilon 1}$)–V381($C_{\gamma 1}$)C	4.7
F9(Benz)–F425(C_ζ)C	3.6				
R22(N_1)–N423(O_1)B	6.2	R22(N_2)–E351(O_2)B	3.0	R22(N_2)–D355(O_1)B	3.5
F23(Benz)–F425(C_ζ)B	5.0				
N24(N_1)–D447(O)B	3.0	N24(N_1)–D377(O)C	3.8	N24(N_1)–D379(O)C	2.9
K25(N_1)–D447(O_1)B	6.1	K25(N_1)–Y379(O_1)A	4.7	K25(N_1)–D379(O)B	2.9
K25(N_1)–N423(O_1)A	5.0				

In contrast to Shaker, Kv1 channels are found to be insensitive to κ-PVIIA [75,76]. This finding can be understood by comparing the binding modes of κ-PVIIA to Shaker and Kv1 channels. Inspection of Table 3 shows that the hydrophobic interactions are missing in the Kv1-κ-PVIIA complexes. A detailed picture of the binding mode in Shaker (Figure 5) helps to explain why. The T449–D447 cross-linking keeps the threonine side chain away from the strongly coupled F9–F425 pair. Indeed the T449Y mutation breaks this cross-linking, which disrupts F9–F425 coupling and renders Shaker insensitive to κ-PVIIA. In a similar fashion, lack of cross-linking in the corresponding residues in Kv1.1 and Kv1.2 prevents the formation of hydrophobic interactions, making them insensitive to κ-PVIIA.

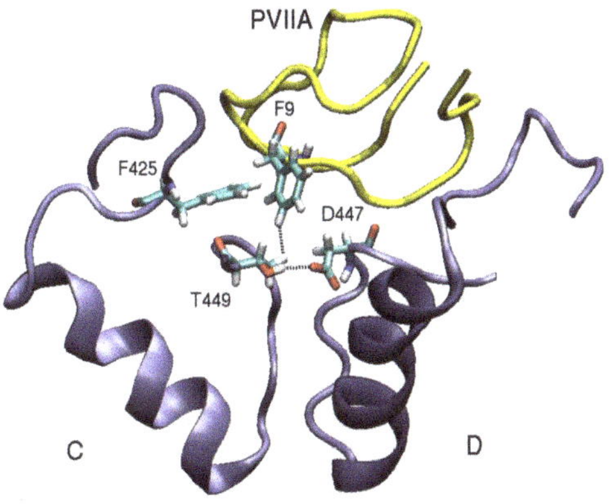

Figure 5. An alternative view of the Shaker-κ-PVIIA complex that demonstrates the importance of the T449–D447 cross-linking in preserving the strong F9–F425 hydrophobic interaction.

4. Sodium Channel Toxins

Computational investigation of sodium channels has just started after the first crystal structure for the bacterial channel NavAb was solved [14]. Two more bacterial Nav channels have been solved since then [84,85]. There have been some earlier model studies of Nav-toxin complexes based on potassium channels and experimental data [86–88], but their accuracy is limited. So far, binding of μ conotoxin to NavAb [56] and scorpion β-toxins to the voltage sensor [58] have been investigated. Due to substantial differences between the bacterial and mammalian Nav channels, homology modelling of the pore domain requires careful validation [89]. Here we briefly discuss binding of μ-conotoxin GIIIA to Nav1.4 to illustrate the differences between the toxin binding modes in potassium and sodium channels (see Figure 6 for the NMR structure of μ-GIIIA). μ-GIIIA is the first conotoxin found to block Nav channels [90], and numerous functional studies of its binding to Nav1.4 have been performed [91–97]. Thus there is a wealth of mutation data to validate the Nav1.4-μ-GIIIA complex models.

A homology model of the pore domain of Nav1.4 was created by aligning the DEKA residues with the corresponding EEEE residues in NavAb. The Nav1.4-μ-GIIIA complex was created using the same procedures as in potassium channel studies. Snapshots of the complex model (Figure 7) shows that μ-GIIIA interacts mainly with the outer ring EEDD residues but has no coupling to the inner ring DEKA residues. R13 makes multiple connections with residues in three domains of Nav1.4 (E403, E758, and D1532), and it is clearly the pore blocking residue, consistent with the mutation experiments [91,92]. K16 is also involved in two interactions (E758 and D1241), again in agreement with the mutation data [87,95,97]. The third important coupling is provided by the K11–D1532 interaction. The proposed model of the Nav1.4-μ-GIIIA complex gives a satisfactory account of the available mutation data. The binding free energy of μ-GIIIA is determined from the PMF calculations and has been found to agree with the experimental value within chemical accuracy. Thus the Nav1.4-μ-GIIIA complex has been well validated and could be used as a template in constructing homology models for the pore domain of other Nav1 channels, which are highly homologous.

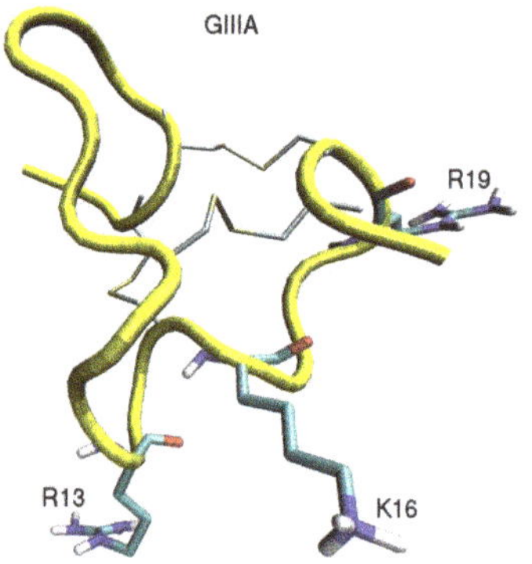

Figure 6. NMR structure of μ-GIIIA [98] showing the important residues involved in binding to Nav1.4.

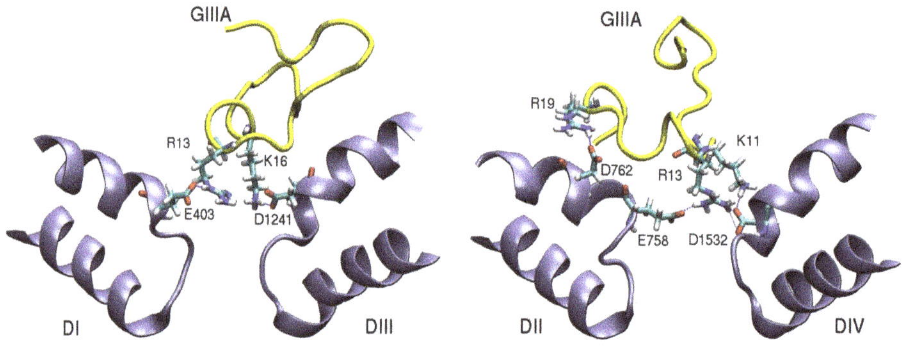

Figure 7. Snapshots of the Nav1.4-μ-GIIIA complex showing the important residues involved in binding. The domains D1–DIII and DII–DIV are shown separately for clarity.

It is of interest to compare the pore domains of the potassium and sodium channels, and point out the differences in toxin binding modes arising from structural constraints. As shown in Figure 8, the selectivity filter in potassium channels is very narrow, long, and has a highly negative potential. This potential attracts a Lys residue (but not the larger Arg) into the filter, which completely blocks the channel. In sodium channels, the selectivity filter is wider and shorter, but the DEKA locus has a smaller negative potential. As a result, toxins preferentially interact with the EEDD residues in the outer ring. Because the outer ring is even wider, only an Arg residue interacting with several domains can completely block the channel—a Lys residue provides only a partial block. The wider opening in sodium channels prevents formation of a tight binding mode observed in many potassium channel-toxin complexes leading to pM affinities. Thus a crucial issue in designing drug leads for sodium channels from toxins is how to increase their relatively low affinities.

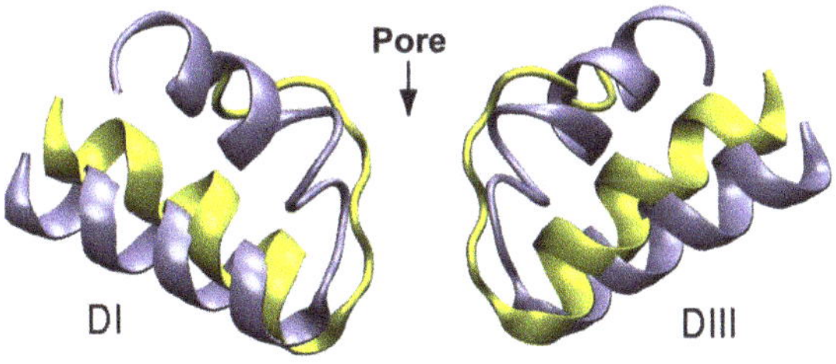

Figure 8. Comparison of the pore domains of Kv1.2 (yellow) and NavAb (blue) channels involved in toxin binding.

5. Conclusions

Rapid advances in computer hardware and software in the last decade has enabled accurate description of the structure and energetics of protein-ligand complexes. As shown in the present work, the accuracy of the computational methods now extends to description of channel-toxin complexes. This opens new avenues for design of drugs from natural sources such as marine toxins. Affinity and selectivity properties of a toxin for a given channel target can be improved by making rational choices for mutations from accurate complex models, and then performing free energy calculations to find the free energy change associated with the mutation. While very good results have been obtained in the examples discussed here, more tests need to be performed to check the predictive power of the computational methods and increase the confidence in them. This is especially so in sodium channels, whose crystal structure has been solved only recently, and there are only a few computational studies of ligand binding to sodium channels as yet. It is expected that there will be a lot of activity in simulation of ligand binding to sodium channels in near future, which will bring our understanding of ligand binding to a level similar to that in potassium channels.

The computational methods have an enormous potential for rational drug design from toxins targeting ion channels, but lack of crystal structures for many types of ion channels is hindering progress. Solution of the structures of channel proteins is the main bottleneck at present and more effort should go in this direction. For example, the ligand-gated ion channels such as nicotinic acetylcholine receptor are even more important therapeutic targets than the voltage-gated ion channels [2], and there are many families of toxins that bind to these channels with high affinity and selectivity. Thus solution of the structures of these channels would enable application of the computational methods for the purpose of designing novel therapeutic agents from the toxin blockers of these channels.

Acknowledgments: This work was supported by grants from the Australian Research Council. Calculations were performed using the HPC facilities at the National Computational Infrastructure (Canberra). We thank Ray Norton for useful discussions on binding properties of ShK toxin and its analogs, and Po-Chia Chen for helping with the simulation studies of toxin binding.

References

1. Hille, B. *Ionic Channels of Excitable Membranes*, 3rd ed.; Sinauer Associates: Sunderland, MA, USA, 2001.
2. Ashcroft, F.M. *Ion Channels and Disease: Channelopathies*; Academic Press: San Diego, CA, USA, 2000.

3. Terlau, H.; Olivera, B.M. Conus venoms: A rich source of novel ion channel-targeted peptides. *Physiol. Rev.* **2004**, *84*, 41–68. [CrossRef]
4. Al-Sabi, A.; McArthur, J.; Ostroumov, V.; French, R.J. Marine toxins that target voltage-gated sodium channels. *Mar. Drugs* **2006**, *4*, 157–192. [CrossRef]
5. Lewis, R.J.; Garcia, M.L. Therapeutic potential of venom peptides. *Nat. Rev. Drug Discov.* **2003**, *2*, 790–802. [CrossRef]
6. French, R.J.; Terlau, H. Sodium channel toxins-receptor targeting and therapeutic potential. *Current Med. Chem.* **2004**, *11*, 3053–3064. [CrossRef]
7. Wulff, H.; Castle, N.A.; Pardo, L.A. Voltage-gated potassium channels as therapeutic targets. *Nat. Rev. Drug Disc.* **2009**, *8*, 982–1001. [CrossRef]
8. Norton, R.S. μ-Conotoxins as leads in the development of new analgesics. *Molecules* **2010**, *15*, 2825–2844. [CrossRef]
9. Beeton, C.; Pennington, M.W.; Norton, R.S. Analogs of the sea anemone potassium channel blocker ShK for the treatment of autoimmune diseases. *Inflamm. Allergy Drug Targets* **2011**, *10*, 313–321. [CrossRef]
10. Chi, V.; Pennington, M.W.; Norton, R.S.; Tarcha, E.J.; Londono, L.M.; Sims-Fahey, B.; Upadhyay, S.K.; Lakey, J.T.; Iadonato, S.; Wulff, H.; *et al.* Development of a sea anemone toxin as an immunomodulator for therapy of autoimmune diseases. *Toxicon* **2012**, *59*, 529–546. [CrossRef]
11. Doyle, D.A.; Cabral, J.M.; Pfuetzner, R.A.; Kuo, A.; Gulbis, J.M.; Cohen, S.L.; Chait, B.T.; MacKinnon, R. The structure of the potassium channel: Molecular basis of K^+ conduction and selectivity. *Science* **1998**, *280*, 69–77. [CrossRef]
12. MacKinnon, R. Potassium channels and the atomic basis of selective ion conduction. *Angew. Chem. Int. Ed.* **2004**, *43*, 4265–4277. [CrossRef]
13. Long, S.B.; Tao, X.; Campbell, E.B.; MacKinnon, R. Atomic structure of a voltage-dependent K^+ channel in a lipid membrane-like environment. *Nature* **2007**, *450*, 376–382. [CrossRef]
14. Payandeh, J.; Scheuer, T.; Zheng, N.; Catterall, W.A. The crystal structure of a voltage-gated sodium channel. *Nature* **2011**, *475*, 353–358. [CrossRef]
15. Pearlman, D.A; Case, D.A.; Caldwell, J.W.; Ross, W.S.; Cheatham, T.E.; DeBolt, S.; Ferguson, D.; Seibel, G.; Kollman, P.A. AMBER, a package of computer programs for applying molecular mechanics, normal mode analysis, molecular dynamics, and free energy calculations to simulate the structural and energetic properties of molecules. *Comp. Phys. Commun.* **1995**, *91*, 1–41. [CrossRef]
16. MacKerell, A.D., Jr.; Bashford, D.; Bellott, M.; Dunbrack, R.L., Jr.; Evanseck, J.D.; Field, M.J.; Fisher, S.; Gao, J.; Guo, H.; Ha, S.; *et al.* All-atom empirical potential for molecular modeling and dynamics studies of proteins. *J. Phys. Chem. B* **1998**, *102*, 3586–3616. [CrossRef]
17. Lindahl, E.; Hess, B.; van der Spoel, D. GROMACS 3.0: A package for molecular simulation and trajectory analysis. *J. Mol. Model.* **2001**, *7*, 306–317.
18. Alonso, H.; Bliznyuk, A.A.; Gready, J.E. Combining docking and molecular dynamic simulations in drug design. *Med. Res. Rev.* **2006**, *26*, 531–568. [CrossRef]
19. Gilson, M.K.; Zhou, H.X. Calculation of protein-ligand binding energies. *Ann. Rev. Biophys. Biomol. Struct.* **2007**, *36*, 21–42. [CrossRef]
20. Deng, Y.; Roux, B. Computations of standard binding free energies with molecular dynamics simulations. *J. Phys. Chem. B* **2009**, *113*, 2234–2246. [CrossRef]
21. Christ, C.D.; Mark, A.E.; van Gunsteren, W.F. Basic ingredients of free energy calculations. *J. Comput. Chem.* **2010**, *31*, 1569–1582.
22. Steinbrecher, T.; Labahn, A. Towards accurate free energy calculations in ligand-protein binding studies. *Curr. Med. Chem.* **2010**, *17*, 767–785. [CrossRef]
23. Halperin, I.; Ma, B.; Wolfson, H.; Nussinov, R. Principles of docking: An overview of search algorithms and a guide to scoring functions. *Proteins* **2002**, *47*, 409–443. [CrossRef]
24. Brooijmans, N.; Kuntz, I.D. Molecular recognition and docking algorithms. *Ann. Rev. Biophys. Biomol. Struct.* **2003**, *32*, 335–373. [CrossRef]
25. Warren, G.L.; Andrews, C.W.; Capelli, A.M.; Clarke, B.; LaLonde, J.; Lambert, M.H.; Lindvall, M.; Nevins, N.; Semus, S.F.; Senger, S.; *et al.* A critical assessment of docking programs and scoring functions. *J. Med. Chem.* **2006**, *49*, 5912–5931. [CrossRef]

26. Morris, G.M.; Goodsell, D.S.; Halliday, R.S.; Huey, R.; Hart, W.E.; Belew, R.K.; Olson, A.J. Automated docking using a Lamarckian genetic algorithm and empirical binding free energy function. *J. Comput. Chem.* **1998**, *19*, 1639–1662. [CrossRef]
27. Mintseris, J.; Pierce, B.; Wiehe, K.; Anderson, R.; Chen, R.; Weng, Z. Integrating statistical pair potentials into prtotein complex prediction. *Proteins* **2007**, *69*, 511–520. [CrossRef]
28. Patra, S.M.; Bastug, T.; Kuyucak, S. Binding of organic cations to gramicidin: A channel studied with AutoDock and molecular dynamics simulations. *J. Phys. Chem. B* **2007**, *111*, 11303–11311. [CrossRef]
29. Ander, M.; Luzhkov, V.B.; Aqvist, J. Ligand binding to the voltage-gated Kv1.5 potassium channel in the open state—Docking and computer simulations of a homology model. *Biophys. J.* **2007**, *94*, 820–831. [CrossRef]
30. Yi, H.; Qiu, S.; Cao, Z.J.; Wu, Y.L.; Li, W.X. Molecular basis of inhibitory peptide maurotoxin recognizing Kv1.2 channel explored by ZDOCK and molecular dynamic simulations. *Proteins* **2008**, *70*, 844–854.
31. Chen, P.C.; Kuyucak, S. Mechanism and energetics of charybdotoxin unbinding from a potassium channel from molecular dynamics simulations. *Biophys. J.* **2009**, *96*, 2577–2588. [CrossRef]
32. Chen, P.C.; Kuyucak, S. Developing a comparative docking protocol for the prediction of peptide selectivity profiles: Investigation of potassium channel toxins. *Toxins* **2012**, *4*, 110–138. [CrossRef]
33. Yu, L.P.; Sun, C.H.; Song, D.Y.; Shen, J.W.; Xu, N.; Gunasekera, A.; Hajduk, P.J.; Olejniczak, E.T. Nuclear magnetic resonance structural studies of a potassium channel-charybdotoxin complex. *Biochemistry* **2005**, *44*, 15834–15841. [CrossRef]
34. Dominguez, C.; Boelens, R.; Bonvin, A.M. HADDOCK: A protein-protein docking approach based on biochemical or biophysical information. *J. Am. Chem. Soc.* **2003**, *125*, 1731–1737. [CrossRef]
35. De Vries, S.J.; van Dijk, A.D.; Krzeminski, M.; van Dijk, M.; Thureau, A.; Hsu, V.; Wassenaar, T.; Bonvin, A.M. HADDOCK *versus* HADDOCK: New features and performance of HADDOCK2.0 on the CAPRI targets. *Proteins* **2007**, *69*, 726–733. [CrossRef]
36. Bastug, T.; Kuyucak, S. Importance of the peptide backbone description in modeling the selectivity filter in potassium channels. *Biophys. J.* **2009**, *96*, 4006–4012. [CrossRef]
37. Bastug, T.; Kuyucak, S. Comparative study of the energetics of ion permeation in Kv1.2 and KcsA potassium channels. *Biophys. J.* **2011**, *100*, 629–636. [CrossRef]
38. Humphrey, W.; Dalke, A.; Schulten, K. VMD—Visual molecular dynamics. *J. Mol. Graph.* **1996**, *14*, 33–38. [CrossRef]
39. Phillips, J.C.; Braun, R.; Wang, W.; Gumbart, J.; Tajkhorshid, E.; Villa, E.; Chipot, C.; Skeel, R.D.; Kale, L.; Schulten, K. Scalable molecular dynamics with NAMD. *J. Comput. Chem.* **2005**, *26*, 1781–1802. [CrossRef]
40. MacKerell, A.D.; Feig, M.; Brooks, C.L. Extending the treatment of backbone energetics in protein force fields. *J. Comput. Chem.* **2004**, *25*, 1400–1415. [CrossRef]
41. Allen, M.P.; Tildesley, D.J. *Computer Simulation of Liquids*; Oxford University Press: London, UK, 1987.
42. Frenkel, D.; Smit, B. *Understanding Molecular Simulation: From Algorithms to Applications*; Academic Press: San Diego, CA, USA, 1996.
43. Leach, A.R. *Molecular Modelling, Principles, Applications*; Prentice Hall: New York, NY, USA, 2001.
44. Bastug, T.; Kuyucak, S. Molecular dynamics simulations of membrane proteins. *Biophys. Rev.* **2012**, *4*, 271–282. [CrossRef]
45. Woo, H.; Roux, B. Calculation of absolute protein-ligand binding free energy from computer simulations. *Proc. Natl. Acad. Sci. USA* **2005**, *102*, 6825–6830. [CrossRef]
46. Bastug, T.; Kuyucak, S. Energetics of ion permeation, rejection, binding and block in gramicidin: A from free energy simulations. *Biophys. J.* **2006**, *90*, 3941–3950. [CrossRef]
47. Torrie, G.M.; Valleau, J.P. Nonphysical sampling distributions in Monte Carlo free-energy estimation: Umbrella sampling. *J. Comput. Phys.* **1977**, *23*, 187–199. [CrossRef]
48. Kumar, S.; Bouzida, D; Swensen, R.H.; Kollman, P.A.; Rosenberg, J.M. The weighted histogram analysis method for free-energy calculations on biomolecules. *J. Comput. Chem.* **1992**, *13*, 1011–1021. [CrossRef]
49. Jarzynski, C. Nonequilibrium equality for free energy diffrences. *Phys. Rev. Lett.* **1997**, *78*, 2690–2693. [CrossRef]
50. Park, S.; Schulten, K. Calculating potentials of mean force from steered molecular dynamics simulations. *J. Chem. Phys.* **2004**, *120*, 5946–5961. [CrossRef]
51. Bastug, T.; Kuyucak, S. Application of Jarzynski's equality in simple versus complex systems. *Chem. Phys. Lett.* **2007**, *436*, 383–387. [CrossRef]

52. Bastug, T.; Chen, P.C.; Patra, S.M.; Kuyucak, S. Potential of mean force calculations of ligand binding to ion channels from Jarzynski's equality and umbrella sampling. *J. Chem. Phys.* **2008**, *128*, 104–112.
53. Chen, P.C.; Kuyucak, S. Accurate determination of the binding free energy for KcsA-Charybdotoxin complex from the potential of mean force calculations with restraints. *Biophys. J.* **2011**, *100*, 2466–2474. [CrossRef]
54. Khabiri, M.; Nikouee, A.; Cwiklik, L.; Grissmer, S.; Ettrich, R. Charybdotoxin unbinding from the mKv1.3 potassium channel: A combined computational and experimental study. *J. Phys. Chem. B* **2011**, *115*, 11490–11500. [CrossRef]
55. Chen, R.; Robinson, A.; Gordon, D.; Chung, S.H. Modeling the binding of three toxins to the voltage-gated potassium channel (Kv1.3). *Biophys. J.* **2011**, *101*, 2652–2660. [CrossRef]
56. Chen, R.; Chung, S.H. Binding modes of μ-conotoxin to the bacterial sodium channel (NaVAb). *Biophys. J.* **2012**, *102*, 483–488. [CrossRef]
57. Chen, R.; Chung, S.H. Structural basis of the selective block of Kv1.2 by maurotoxin from computer simulations. *PLoS One* **2012**, *7*, e47253.
58. Chen, R.; Chung, S.H. Conserved functional surface of antimammalian scorpion β-toxins. *J. Phys. Chem. B* **2012**, *116*, 4796–4800.
59. Rashid, M.H.; Kuyucak, S. Affinity and selectivity of ShK toxin for the Kv1 potassium channels from free energy simulations. *J. Phys. Chem. B* **2012**, *116*, 4812–4822.
60. Pennington, M.W.; Rashid, M.H.; Tajhya, R.B.; Beeton, C.; Kuyucak, S.; Norton, R.S. A *C*-terminally amidated analogue of ShK is a potent and selective blocker of the voltage-gated potassium channel Kv1.3. *FEBS Lett.* **2012**, *586*, 3996–4001.
61. Mahdavi, S.; Kuyucak, S. Why drosophila shaker K^+ channel is not a good model for ligand binding to voltage-gated Kv1 channels. *Biochemistry* **2013**, in press.
62. Beveridge, D.L.; DiCapua, F.M. Free energy via molecular simulation: Applications to chemi-cal and biomolecular systems. *Annu. Rev. Biophys. Biophys. Chem.* **1989**, *18*, 431–492.
63. Heinzelmann, G.; Bastug, T.; Kuyucak, S. Free energy simulations of ligand binding to the aspartate transporter GltPh. *Biophys. J.* **2011**, *101*, 2380–2388.
64. Huang, X.; Dong, F.; Zhou, H.X. Electrostatic recognition and induced fit in the κ-PVIIA toxin binding to Shaker potassium channel. *J. Am. Chem. Soc.* **2005**, *127*, 6836–6849.
65. Tudor, J.E.; Pallaghy, P.K.; Pennington, M.W.; Norton, R.S. Solution structure of ShK toxin, a novel potassium channel inhibitor from a sea anemone. *Nat. Struct. Biol.* **1996**, *3*, 317–320.
66. Scanlon, M.J.; Naranjo, D.; Thomas, L.; Alewood, P.F.; Lewis, R.J.; Craik, D.J. Solution structure and proposed binding mechanism of a novel potassium channel toxin kappa-conotoxin PVIIA. *Structure* **1997**, *5*, 1585–1597.
67. Wulff, H.; Calabresi, P.A.; Allie, R.; Yun, S.; Pennington, M.; Beeton, C.; Chandy, K.G. The voltage-gated Kv1.3 K^+ channel in effector memory T cells as new target for MS. *J. Clin. Invest.* **2003**, *111*, 1703–1713.
68. Beeton, C.; Wulff, H.; Standifer, N.E.; Azam, P.; Mullen, K.M.; Pennington, M.W.; Kolski-Andreaco, A.; Wei, E.; Grino, A.; Counts, D.R.; *et al.* Kv1.3 channels are a therapeutic target for T cell-mediated autoimmune diseases. *Proc. Natl. Acad. Sci. USA* **2006**, *103*, 17414–17419.
69. Castaneda, O.; Sotolongo, V; Amor, A.M.; Stocklin, R.; Anderson, A.J.; Harvey, A.L.; Engstrom, A.; Wernstedt, C.; Karlsson, E. Characterization of a potassium channel toxin from the Caribbean Sea anemone *Stichodactyla helianthus*. *Toxicon* **1995**, *33*, 603–613.
70. Pohl, J.; Hubalek, F.; Byrnes, M.E.; Nielsen, K.R.; Woods, A.; Pennington, M.W. Assignment of the three disulfide bonds in ShK toxin, a potent potassium channel blocker from the sea anemone Stichodactyla helianthus. *Lett. Pept. Sci.* **1994**, *1*, 291–297.
71. Kalman, K.; Pennington, M.W.; Lanigan, M.D.; Nguyen, A.; Rauer, H.; Mahnir, V.; Paschetto, K.; Kem, W.R.; Grissmer, S.; Gutman, G.A. ShK-Dap22, a potent Kv1.3-specific immunosuppressive polypeptide. *J. Biol. Chem.* **1998**, *273*, 32697–32707.
72. Beeton, C.; Pennington, M.; Wulf, H.; Singh, S.; Nugent, D.; Crossley, G.; Khaytin, I.; Calabresi, P.A.; Chen, C.Y.; Gutman, G.A.; Chandy, K.G. Targeting effector memory T cells with a selective peptide inhibitor of Kv1.3 channels for therapy of autoimmune diseases. *Mol. Pharmacol.* **2005**, *67*, 1369–1381.
73. Pennington, M.W.; Beeton, C.; Galea, C.A.; Smith, B.J.; Chi, V.; Monaghan, K.P.; Garcia, A.; Rangaraju, S.; Giuffrida, A.; Plank, D.; *et al.* Engineering a stable and selective peptide blocker of the Kv1.3.3 channel in T lymphocytes. *Mol. Pharmacol.* **2009**, *75*, 762–773.

74. Rauer, H.; Pennington, M.; Cahalan, M.; Chandy, K.G. Structural conservation of the pores of calcium-activated and voltage-gated potassium channels determined by a sea anemone toxin. *J. Biol. Chem.* **1999**, *274*, 21885–21892.
75. Terlau, H.; Shon, K.J.; Grilley, M.; Stocker, M.; Stuhmer, W.; Olivera, B.M. Strategy for rapid immobilization of prey by a fish-hunting marine snail. *Nature* **1996**, *381*, 148–151.
76. Shon, K.J.; Stocker, M.; Terlau, H.; Stuhmer, W.; Jacobsen, R.; Walker, C.; Grilley, M.; Watkins, M.; Hillyard, D.R.; Gray, W.R.; Olivera, B.M. κ-Conotoxin PVIIA is a peptide inhibiting the Shaker K^+ channel. *J. Biol. Chem.* **1998**, *273*, 33–38.
77. Jacobsen, R.B.; Koch, E.D.; Lange-Malecki, B.; Stocker, M.; Verhey, J.; van Wagoner, R.M.; Vyazovkina, A.; Olivera, B.M.; Terlau, H. Single amino acid substitutions in *κ*-conotoxin PVIIA disrupt interaction with the Shaker K^+ channel. *J. Biol. Chem.* **2000**, *275*, 24639–24644.
78. Garcia, E.; Scanlon, M.; Naranjo, D. A marine snail neurotoxin shares with scorpion toxins a convergn et mechanism of blockade on the pore of voltage-gated K channels. *J. Gen. Physiol.* **1999**, *114*, 141–157.
79. Terlau, H.; Boccaccio, A.; Olivera, B.M.; Conti, F. The block of Shaker K^+ channels by *κ*-conotoxin PVIIA is state dependent. *J. Gen. Physiol.* **1999**, *114*, 125–140.
80. Boccaccio, A.; Conti, F.; Olivera, B.M.; Terlau, H. Binding of *κ*-conotoxin PVIIA to Shaker K^+ channels reveals different K^+ and Rb^+ occupancies with the ion channel pore. *J. Gen. Physiol.* **2004**, *124*, 71–81.
81. Olivia, C.; Gonzalez, V.; Naranjo, D. Slow inactivation in voltage gated potassium channels is insensitive to the binding of pore occluding peptide toxins. *Biophys. J.* **2005**, *89*, 1009–1019.
82. Jouirou, B.; Mouhat, S.; Andreotti, N.; de Waard, M.; Sabatier, J.M. Toxin determinants required for interaction with voltage-gated K^+ channels. *Toxicon* **2004**, *43*, 909–914.
83. Rodriguez de la Vega, R.C.; Possani, L.D. Current views on scorpion toxins specific for K^+-channels. *Toxicon* **2004**, *43*, 865–875.
84. Zhang, X.; Ren, W.; DeCaen, P.; Yan, C.; Tao, X.; Tang, L.; Wang, J.; Hasegawa, K.; Kumasaka, T.; He, J.; *et al.* Crystal structure of an orthologue of the NaChBac voltage-gated sodium channel. *Nature* **2012**, *486*, 130–134.
85. Payandeh, J.; Scheuer, T.; Zheng, N.; Catterall, W.A. Crystal structure of a voltage-gated sodium channel in two potentially inactivated states. *Nature* **2012**, *486*, 135–139.
86. Tikhonov, D.B.; Zhorov, B.S. Modeling P-loops domain of sodium channel: Homology with potassium channels and interaction with ligands. *Biophys. J.* **2005**, *88*, 184–197. [CrossRef]
87. Choudhary, G.; Aliste, M.P.; Tieleman, D.P.; French, R.J.; Dudley, S.C., Jr. Docking of *μ*-conotoxin GIIIA in the sodium channel outer vestibule. *Channels* **2007**, *1*, 344–352.
88. Fozzard, H.A.; Lipkind, G.M. The tetrodotoxin binding site is within the outer vestibule of the sodium channel. *Mar. Drugs* **2010**, *8*, 219–234.
89. Tikhonov, D.B.; Zhorov, B.S. Architecture and pore block of eukaryotic voltage-gated sodium channels in view of NavAb bacterial sodium channel structure. *Mol. Pharmacol.* **2012**, *82*, 97–104.
90. Cruz, L.J.; Gray, W.R.; Olivera, B.M.; Zeikus, R.D.; Kerr, L.; Yoshikami, D.; Moczydlowski, E. Conus geographus toxins that discriminate between neuronal and muscle sodium channels. *J. Biol. Chem.* **1985**, *260*, 9280–9288.
91. Sato, K.; Ishida, Y.; Wakamatsu, K.; Kato, R.; Honda, H.; Ohizumi, Y.; Nakamura, H.; Ohya, M.; Lancelin, J.M.; Kohda, D.; *et al.* Active site of *μ*-conotoxin GIIIA, a peptide blocker of muscle sodium channels. *J. Biol. Chem.* **1991**, *266*, 16989–16991.
92. Becker, S.; Prusak-Sochaczewski, E.; Zamponi, G.; Beck-Sickinger, A.G.; Gordon, R.D.; French, R.J. Action of derivatives of *μ*-conotoxin GIIIA on sodium channels. *Biochemistry* **1992**, *31*, 8229–8238.
93. Chang, N.S.; French, R.J.; Lipkind, G.M.; Fozzard, H.A.; Dudley, S., Jr. Predominant interactions between *μ*-conotoxin Arg-13 and the skeletal muscle Na+ channel localized by mutant cycle analysis. *Biochemistry* **1998**, *37*, 4407–4419.
94. Dudley, S.C., Jr.; Chang, N.; Hall, J.; Lipkind, G.; Fozzard, H.A.; French, R.J. *μ*-Conotoxin GIIIA interactions with the voltage-gated Na^+ channel predict a clockwise arrangement of the domains. *J. Gen. Physiol.* **2000**, *116*, 679–690.
95. Li, R.A.; Ennis, I.L.; French, R.J.; Dudley, S.C., Jr.; Tomaselli, G.F.; Marban, E. Clockwise domain arrangement of the sodium channel revealed by *μ*-conotoxin (GIIIA) docking orientation. *J. Biol. Chem.* **2001**, *276*, 11072–11077.

96. Hui, K.; Lipkind, G.; Fozzard, H.A.; French, R.J. Electrostatic and steric contributions to block of the skeletal muscle sodium channel by μ-conotoxin. *J. Gen. Physiol.* **2002**, *119*, 45–54.
97. Xue, T.; Ennis, I.L.; Sato, K.; French, R.J.; Li, R.A. Novel interactions identified between μ-conotoxin and the Na+ channel domain I P-loop: Implications for toxin-pore binding geometry. *Biophys. J.* **2003**, *85*, 2299–2310.
98. Wakamatsu, K.; Kohda, D.; Hatanaka, H.; Lancelin, J.M.; Ishida, Y.; Oya, M.; Nakamura, H.; Inagaki, F.; Sato, K. Structure-activity relationships of μ-conotoxin GIIIA: Structure determination of active and inactive sodium channel blocker peptides by NMR and simulated annealing calculations. *Biochemistry* **1992**, *31*, 12577–12584.

marine drugs

MDPI

Article

Salternamide A Suppresses Hypoxia-Induced Accumulation of HIF-1α and Induces Apoptosis in Human Colorectal Cancer Cells

Duc-Hiep Bach, Seong-Hwan Kim, Ji-Young Hong, Hyen Joo Park, Dong-Chan Oh and Sang Kook Lee *

College of Pharmacy, Seoul National University, Seoul 151-742, Korea; bdhiep90@snu.ac.kr (D.-H.B.); yanberk@snu.ac.kr (S.-H.K.); jyhong7876@daum.net (J.-Y.H.); phj00@snu.ac.kr (H.J.P.); dongchanoh@snu.ac.kr (D.-C.O.)

* Author to whom correspondence should be addressed; sklee61@snu.ac.kr (S.K.L.); Tel.: +82-2-880-2475; Fax: +82-2-762-8322.

Academic Editor: Sylvia Urban
Received: 28 August 2015; Accepted: 12 November 2015; Published: 19 November 2015

Abstract: Hypoxia inducible factor-1α (HIF-1α) is an essential regulator of the cellular response to low oxygen concentrations, activating a broad range of genes that provide adaptive responses to oxygen deprivation. HIF-1α is overexpressed in various cancers and therefore represents a considerable chemotherapeutic target. Salternamide A (SA), a novel small molecule that is isolated from a halophilic *Streptomyces* sp., is a potent cytotoxic agent against a variety of human cancer cell lines. However, the mechanisms by which SA inhibits tumor growth remain to be elucidated. In the present study, we demonstrate that SA efficiently inhibits the hypoxia-induced accumulation of HIF-1α in a time- and concentration-dependent manner in various human cancer cells. In addition, SA suppresses the upstream signaling of HIF-1α, such as PI3K/Akt/mTOR, p42/p44 MAPK, and STAT3 signaling under hypoxic conditions. Furthermore, we found that SA induces cell death by stimulating G2/M cell cycle arrest and apoptosis in human colorectal cancer cells. Taken together, SA was identified as a novel small molecule HIF-1α inhibitor from marine natural products and is potentially a leading candidate in the development of anticancer agents.

Keywords: salternamide A (SA); HIF-1α; PI3K/Akt/mTOR; p42/p44 MAPK; STAT3; cell death

1. Introduction

The transcription factor hypoxia-inducible factor-1 (HIF-1) plays a pivotal role in regulating the initiation of genes that are involved in decisive aspects of cancer biology, such as angiogenesis, cell survival, differentiation, invasion, tumor progression, and glucose metabolism [1–6]. HIF-1 is a heterodimer that consists of HIF-1α and HIF-1β subunits. In addition, HIF-1 activity in tumors depends on the availability of the HIF-1α subunit and the levels of HIF-1α expression under hypoxic conditions [4]. Indeed, HIF-1α is overexpressed in a variety of human cancers compared to normal tissues [7,8]. Consequently, HIF-1α is an appealing intracellular target for treating a wide range of hypoxia-related pathologies by targeted cancer therapy [9].

The overexpression of HIF-1α is due to the fundamental interaction between various metabolic pathways and factors that lead to particular genetic alterations and extracellular stimuli, such as hypoxia that impact both protein degradation and synthesis [10]. Two main signaling pathways are involved in the regulation of HIF-1α function and protein levels: the phosphatidylinositol 3-kinase (PI3K) and the mitogen-activated protein kinase (MAPK) pathways [4]. Signaling from the PI3K pathway enhances HIF-1α synthesis through the mammalian target of the rapamycin protein complex (mTOR; a kinase that functions downstream of PI3K and Akt), likely by heightening HIF-1α translation. The p42/p44 MAPK pathway may induce the transactivation function of HIF-1α through the direct phosphorylation of HIF-1α [11] or by upregulating its cofactor p300 [12]. Additionally, recent studies have reported that the signal transducer and activator of transcription-3 (STAT3) is activated in response to hypoxia, a common feature of various solid tumors [13,14]. Activated STAT3 also mediates the upregulation of HIF-1α by enhancing its transcriptional activity [15].

Salternamide A (SA), a novel small molecule marine agent, was recently isolated by our group from a halophilic *Streptomyces* sp. possessing anti-proliferative activity against various cancer cells [16]. SA was identified as the first secondary metabolite from a saltern-derived actinomycetes microorganism and the first chlorinated member of the manumycin family. However, there has been no report further evaluating its anticancer activity and mechanisms of action in human colon cancer cells.

In the present study, we attempted to investigate the mechanism by which SA suppresses HIF-1α protein accumulation and induces cell death in HCT116 human colon cancer cells.

2. Results and Discussion

2.1. Salternamide A Suppresses Hypoxia-Induced HIF-1α Protein Accumulation in Various Cancer Cells

To investigate whether SA (Figure 1A) affects HIF-1α induced by hypoxia, HCT116 cells were exposed to normoxic or hypoxic ($CoCl_2$ treatment) conditions for 2, 4, 8, 12, or 24 h in the presence of 10 μM SA. As shown in Figure 1B, HIF-1α expression was significantly induced by hypoxia-mimetic $CoCl_2$ treatment, starting from as early as 4 h. However, SA effectively suppressed hypoxia-induced HIF-1α protein expression at 8 h along with marked suppression at 12 and 24 h (Figure 1B). In addition, when treated with SA for 8 h under hypoxic conditions, SA suppressed the accumulation of hypoxia-induced HIF-1α protein in a concentration-dependent manner (Figure 1C).

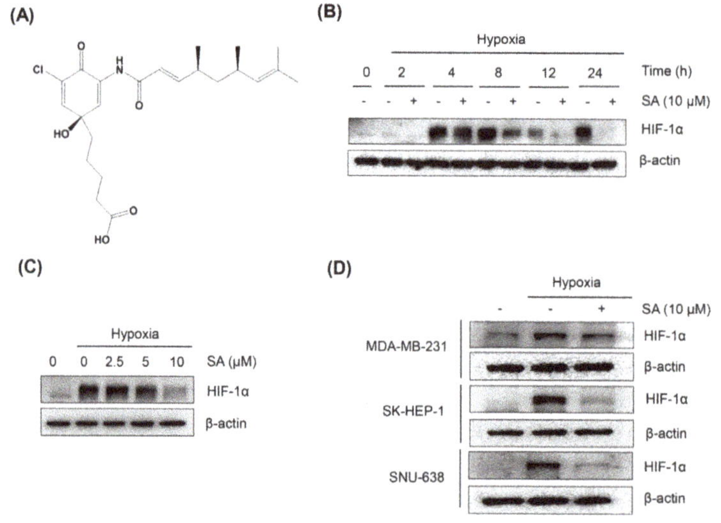

Figure 1. Effect of SA on hypoxia-induced HIF-1α protein accumulation in various cancer cells. (**A**) Chemical structure of SA; (**B**) HCT116 cells were treated at the indicated time points under normoxic or hypoxic conditions ($CoCl_2$ treatment) in the presence or absence of SA (10 μM); (**C**) HCT116 cells were treated for 8 h under normoxic or hypoxic conditions in the presence or absence of increasing SA concentrations; (**D**) MDA-MB-231, SK-HEP-1, and SNU-638 cells were treated with 10 μM SA for 8 h under normoxic or hypoxic conditions. Immunoblotting analysis was performed to determine HIF-1α and β-actin protein levels.

To further examine whether the suppressive effect of SA on HIF-1α expression is applicable to a variety of cancer cell lines with different genetic backgrounds (wild-type or mutated p53), given that HIF-1α is destabilized by p53 [17] in different organs, SK-HEP-1 (liver), SNU-638 (gastric), and MDA-MB-231 (breast) cancer cells were treated with 10 μM SA for 8 h. SA effectively suppressed the expression of HIF-1α in the tested cancer cells, similar to the results shown in HCT116 cells (Figure 1D). These findings suggest that SA suppresses HIF-1α expression in various cancer cell types by blocking HIF-1α protein accumulation in response to hypoxic conditions.

2.2. Suppression of HIF-1α Accumulation by Salternamide A in HCT116 Cells Is Independent of Proteasomal Degradation

In general, the accumulation of HIF-1α depends on the balance between its degradation and synthesis (translation) [18]. To determine whether SA is able to suppress HIF-1α protein accumulation by promoting its degradation, the cells were pretreated with the proteasome inhibitor MG132, followed by SA treatment in HCT116 cells. As shown in Figure 2A, pretreatment with MG132 resulted in the accumulation of HIF-1α, but SA efficiently abrogated the accumulation of HIF-1α despite proteasome suppression, indicating that SA decreases HIF-1α protein accumulation through a pathway independent of proteasomal degradation.

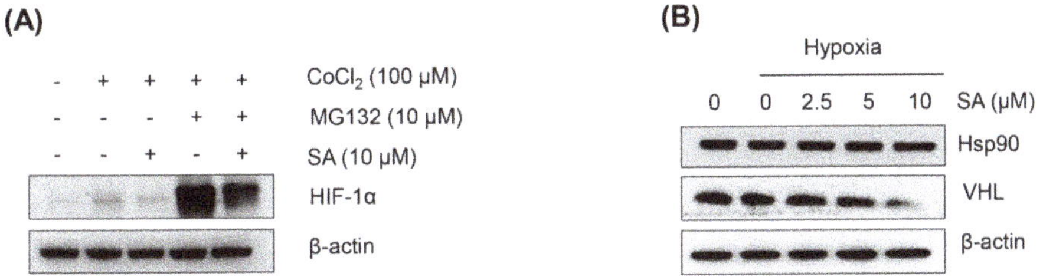

Figure 2. Effect of SA on the degradation of HIF-1α. (**A**) HCT116 cells were treated with a proteasome inhibitor (10 μM MG132) and 10 μM SA under normoxic or hypoxic conditions before immunoblotting; (**B**) for VHL and Hsp90 immunoblotting, HCT116 cells were treated with SA and cultured for 8 h under normoxic or hypoxic conditions, respectively.

The von Hippel-Lindau (VHL) tumor suppressor protein recruits an E3-ubiquitin ligase that targets HIF-1α for proteasomal degradation [4]. In addition, heat-shock protein 90 (Hsp90) binds to HIF-1α and promotes its stability [19]. To determine whether the suppression of HIF-1α protein expression by SA is associated with these adaptor proteins, Western blot analysis was performed under hypoxic conditions with the treatment of SA in HCT116 cells. As a result, SA did not significantly enhance the VHL or abrogate Hsp90 expression in the HCT116 cells (Figure 2B). These data suggest that the suppression of HIF-1α accumulation by SA under hypoxic conditions might not be associated with the enhancement of the degradation of HIF-1α under these conditions. Further study revealed that SA did not affect HIF-1α gene transcription or HIF-1α mRNA stability (data not shown). Overall, the suppressive effect of SA on the accumulation of HIF-1α protein expression under hypoxic conditions might be due in part to the downregulation of the translation of HIF-1α mRNA. These translational regulations should be further clarified in detail.

2.3. Salternamide A Suppresses the Hypoxia-Induced Accumulation of HIF-1α via the Regulation of Signal Transduction Pathways

Recent studies have reported that the PI3K/Akt/mTOR and p42/p44 MAPK pathways are associated with the regulation of HIF-1α protein synthesis at the translational level [10,20]. The p42/p44 MAPK also enhances the transcriptional activity of HIF-1α [11]. To address the potential involvement of these pathways in the SA-mediated suppression of HIF-1α accumulation, the expression of the proteins in the signal transduction pathway was determined by Western blot analysis. As shown in Figure 3A, activated (phosphorylated form) PI3K, Akt, mTOR, and RPS6 expression under hypoxic conditions was downregulated by the treatment of SA (10 μM) in a time-dependent manner. A subsequent study also revealed that SA effectively suppressed the expressions of these signaling proteins in a concentration-dependent manner (Figure 3B). In addition, SA also downregulated the activation of p70S6K1 (Thr^{389}), 4E-BP1 ($Thr^{37/46}$), eIF4E (Ser^{209}), and RPS6 ($Ser^{235/236}$), which are downstream target molecules of mTOR complex 1 (mTORC1) signaling pathways. Therefore, these data suggest that the suppression of HIF-1α protein expression by SA might be partly associated with the downregulation of mTORC1 signaling pathways under hypoxic conditions.

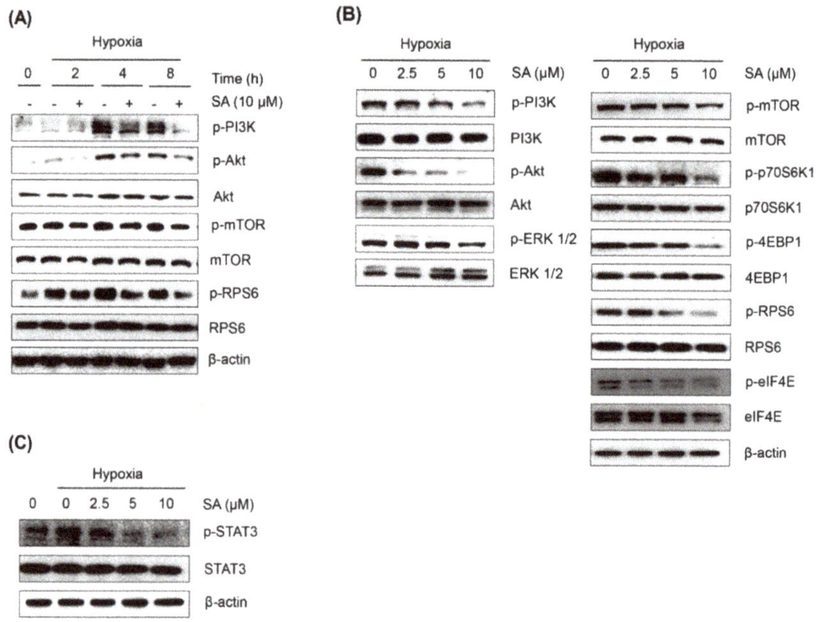

Figure 3. Effect of SA on hypoxia-response protein expressions. (**A**) HCT116 cells were treated at the indicated time points under normoxic or hypoxic conditions in the presence or absence of SA (10 μM) before immunoblotting. (**B** and **C**) HCT116 cells were treated for 8 h under normoxic or hypoxic conditions in the presence or absence of increasing SA concentrations.

Recent reports have also revealed that the transcription factor STAT3 is involved in the transcriptional regulation of HIF-1α and that the activation of STAT3 activity is enhanced by hypoxia [21,22]. In the present study, we also found that hypoxia enhanced STAT3 activation (phosphorylated at the Tyr^{705} residue), and this effect was abrogated by the treatment of SA in a concentration-dependent manner (Figure 3C).

Overall, these findings suggest that the suppression of the PI3K/Akt/mTOR, p42/p44 MAPK, and STAT3 signaling pathways by SA might be associated, in part, with the downregulation of HIF-1α protein synthesis.

2.4. Salternamide A Induces Apoptotic Cell Death in Human Colorectal Cancer Cells

A previous study revealed the anti-proliferative activity of SA in a panel of cancer cell lines [16]. To further elucidate the mechanism of action of the anti-proliferative activity of SA, the effect of SA on the regulation of the cell cycle was determined in HCT116 cells. When treated with SA for 72 h, SA primarily inhibited the growth of HCT116 cells in a concentration-dependent manner (Figure 4A). SA (10 μM) increased the cell population in the sub-G1 phase at 48 h (Figure 4B, right panel). To further elucidate whether cell cycle arrest is associated with the regulation of cell cycle checkpoint proteins, the expression of G2/M cell cycle regulatory proteins was analyzed by Western blotting. As shown in Figure 4C, the expression of p-CDC25C (Ser^{216}), CDC25C, p-CDC2 (Thr^{161}), CDC2, cyclin B1, and cyclin A were significantly suppressed, but the levels of p-chk1 (Ser^{345}) and p-chk2 (Thr^{168}) were upregulated by the treatment of SA. These findings suggest that the anti-proliferative activity of SA is associated, in part, with the induction of the G2/M phase cell cycle arrest by modulating cell cycle regulators in HCT116 cells.

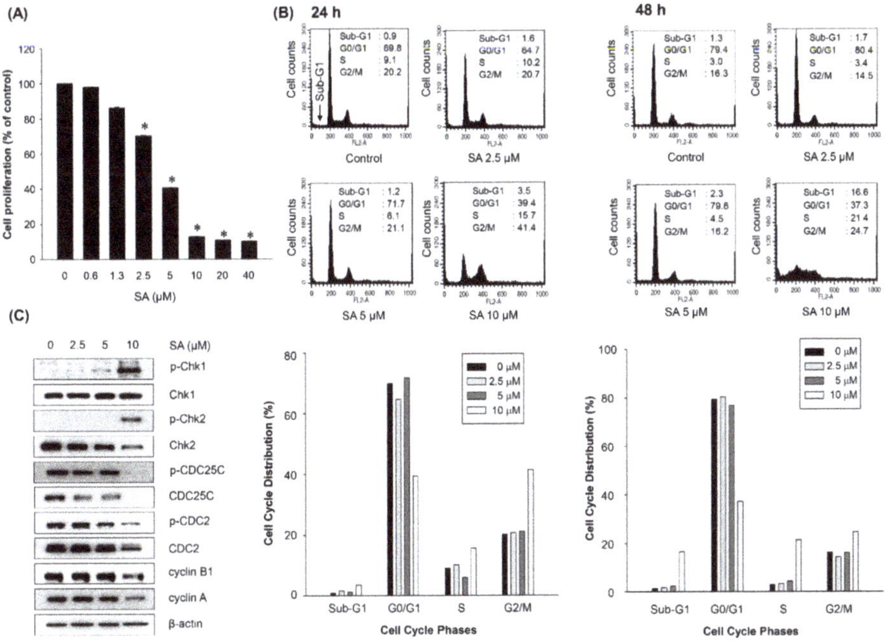

Figure 4. Effect of SA on cell cycle distribution in HCT116 human colorectal cancer cells. (**A**) Anti-proliferative effect of SA on HCT116 cells. HCT116 cells were treated with various concentrations of SA for 72 h, and cell proliferation was determined with the SRB assay. The data represent the mean percentage ± SD compared to the DMSO-treated control group. Each experiment was performed in triplicate (n = 3). * $p < 0.05$ compared with the control group. (**B**) HCT116 cells were treated with SA for 24 or 48 h. The cell cycle distribution was analyzed by flow cytometry. (**C**) Effects of SA on the expression of cell cycle-related proteins in HCT116 colorectal cancer cells. HCT116 cells (2×10^5 cells/mL) were treated with SA for 24 h. Subsequently, the protein expression levels of cell cycle-related proteins were analyzed by Western blotting.

To further confirm whether the induction of the sub-G1 peak by SA (10 μM) at 48 h is related to apoptotic cell death, the cells were treated with SA (10 μM) for 48 h, and the quantification of Annexin-V/PI staining, a marker for apoptosis, was determined by flow cytometry. The number of cells that were positive for the double staining of Annexin-V/PI was significantly increased by SA treatment, suggesting that SA is able to induce apoptotic cell death in cancer cells (Figure 5A). To further unveil the mechanism of SA-induced apoptosis in HCT116 cells, the expression of apoptosis-associated proteins was analyzed by Western blotting. As shown in Figure 5B,C, the expression of cleaved caspase-8, cleaved caspase-3, and cleaved PARP was upregulated, but the expression of pro-caspase-8, caspase-3, pro-PARP, Bcl-2 and Bcl-xL was downregulated in a time- and concentration-dependent manner. In addition, LC3-II is an autophagy-specific marker, and LC3-II formation (LC3 lipidation) is also a key step in autophagy-associated cell death [23]. To evaluate whether the cytotoxic activity of SA is related, in part, to the induction of autophagy, the expression level of LC3-II was determined by 48 h of SA (10 μM) treatment. SA also significantly induced the expression of LC3-II in a time- and concentration-dependent manner. Taken together, these results suggest that the anti-proliferative activity of SA might be due, in part, to the G2/M phase cell cycle arrest and the induction of apoptosis and autophagic cell death in HCT116 cells.

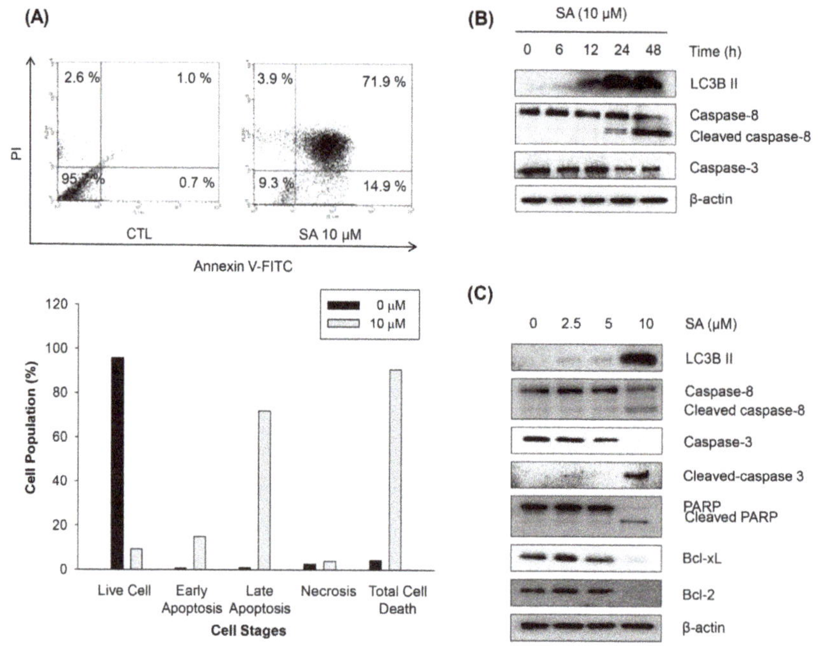

Figure 5. Effects of SA on apoptosis and autophagy in HCT116 human colorectal cancer cells. (**A**) HCT116 cells (1×10^5 cells/mL) were treated with SA for 48 h. Following treatment, HCT116 cells were harvested and stained with Annexin V-FITC and PI and analyzed using flow cytometry as described in the experimental section. (**B**) HCT116 cells were treated at the indicated time points in the presence or absence of SA (10 μM) prior to Western blotting. (**C**) Effects of SA on the expression of apoptosis- and autophagy-related proteins in HCT116 colorectal cancer cells. HCT116 cells (2×10^5 cells/mL) were treated with SA for 48 h; subsequently, the protein expression levels of apoptosis- and autophagy-related proteins were analyzed by Western blotting.

2.5. Discussion

Many efforts have been designed to identify and develop new small molecule HIF-1α inhibitors. Natural products have played an important role in drug discovery and development by providing novel chemical entities. In the present study, we found that salternamide A (SA) is a novel HIF-1α inhibitor derived from natural sources. SA is one of the salternamides that we recently isolated from a halophilic *Streptomyces* sp. of saltern-derived actinomycetes [16]. In terms of chemical characteristics, SA is novel and is the first chlorinated member of the manumycin class. Initially, SA exhibited the most potent cytotoxicity among the isolated salternamides against a panel of cancer cell lines [16]. However, the precise mechanism of action of the anti-proliferative activity of SA is not fully understood. Based on the unique chemical structure and potent growth inhibition of cancer cells, we attempted to elucidate its mechanism of action in cancer cells. From the initial analysis of chemical structures of salternamides with the amide-side chain, we assumed that HIF-1α should be a candidate target molecule. As a result, SA suppressed the accumulation of the HIF-1α protein under hypoxic conditions in human colorectal HCT116 cancer cells.

VHL is the substrate recognition component of an E3 ubiquitin ligase complex that targets HIF-1α and HIF-2α for ubiquitin-mediated degradation under normoxic conditions. The interaction of pVHL (the protein transcript of the VHL gene) with HIF-1α is one of several O_2-dependent events thought to regulate HIF activity [24]. Inactivation of the VHL gene is correlated to the development of highly vascularized tumors. pVHL directs the polyubiquitylation of HIF-1α for ubiquitin-mediated degradation in an oxygen-dependent manner. Therefore, loss of VHL is sufficient not only to stabilize HIF-1α subunits under normoxia, but also to fully activate HIF-mediated responses [24]. Maranchie *et al.* [25], however, reported that loss of the tumor suppressor VHL did not enhance the growth of subcutaneous tumors derived from primary cells. In the present study, the level of VHL was decreased by SA at 10 μM, suggesting that the inhibition of HIF-1α accumulation by SA under hypoxic conditions might not be correlated to the increasing of the degradation of HIF-1α. However, the detailed mechanisms of this action need to be further clarified. Further study revealed that the suppressive effect of SA on the accumulation of HIF-1α might be partly due to the inhibition of the translation of HIF-1α, without affecting the expression level of HIF-1α mRNA or the degradation of the HIF-1α protein.

The expression of HIF-1α is closely regulated by both its protein synthesis and degradation. The translation of HIF-1α is promoted by the axis of mTOR signaling through the activation of p70S6K, 4E-BP1, and eIF4E [26]. The PI3K/Akt/mTOR and p42/p44 MAPK pathways also activate translational regulatory proteins, including 4E-BP1, eIF4E, and p60S6K [4]. SA modulates the mTOR signaling pathways and the axis of PI3K/Akt/MAPK-mediated downstream signaling, thus leading to the suppression HIF-1α translation under hypoxic conditions in cancer cells.

Recent studies have also reported that STAT3 is activated in response to hypoxia in various cancers [13,14], and STAT3 signaling is required for HIF-1α protein accumulation in the activation of endogenous HIF-1α target genes [27,28]. In the present study, SA suppressed the activation of STAT3, which led to the downregulation of HIF-1α protein expression under hypoxic conditions. These findings also suggest that the regulation of STAT3 by SA is partly involved in the suppression of HIF-1α accumulation under hypoxic conditions in cancer cells.

Taken together, although further detailed study is needed to elucidate how the translation of HIF-1α is regulated, SA is considered a novel inhibitor of HIF-1α protein synthesis under hypoxic conditions in cancer cells.

In addition, the anti-proliferative activity of SA was associated with G2/M cell cycle arrest and subsequent apoptotic cell death in HCT116 cancer cells. G2/M phase arrest was highly correlated with the downregulation of CDC25C and CDC2 checkpoint protein expression [27]. The progression from G2 to M phase is regulated by a number of cyclin family members, such as cyclin B1 and CDC2. Cyclin B1, together with cyclin A, promotes the G2/M transition [29,30]. Meanwhile, CDC2 is crucial for the G1/S and G2/M phase transitions of the eukaryotic cell cycle. The phosphatase activity of CDC25C is also implicated in the regulation of the progression of G2/M phase [31]. Chk1 (Checkpoint Kinase 1) and Chk2 (Checkpoint Kinase 2) are multi-functional protein kinases that coordinate the response to specific types of DNA damage [32]. As a result, we found that SA-mediated G2/M phase cell cycle arrest was associated with the regulation of CDC25C and CDC2 and its related checkpoint kinases Chk1/2.

Apoptosis is one of the main types of programmed cell death, and many anti-cancer agents induce apoptosis against cancer cells to achieve therapeutic efficacy [33,34]. We also found that longer and higher concentrations of SA exposure are able to induce apoptotic cell death in the HCT116 cells. Apoptotic cell death by SA was confirmed by significant increases in the proteolytic cleavage of caspase-8, -3 and PARP, and the downregulation of the antiapoptotic Bcl-2 and Bcl-xL proteins.

Autophagy plays a complex role in cancer development, with a tumor-progressive or a tumor-suppressive effect [35]. Apoptosis and autophagy may be interconnected, either antagonistically or cooperatively, in response to various anti-cancer therapeutics in different cancer cells [36]. Herein, we observed that the formation of LC3-II, a marker of autophagy, was also induced by SA, suggesting that autophagy-mediated cell death is also involved in the anti-proliferative activity of SA in HCT116 cancer cells.

3. Materials and Methods

3.1. Materials

Salternamide A (SA, Figure 1A) was dissolved in 100% DMSO and stored at −20 °C for subsequent analysis. Cobalt (II) chloride ($CoCl_2$) and MG132 were purchased from Sigma-Aldrich (St. Louis, MO, USA). Antibodies for HIF-1α, Akt, phospho-Akt (Thr^{308}), PI3K, phospho-PI3K ($Tyr^{458/199}$), RPS6, phospho-RPS6 ($Ser^{235/236}$), p70S6K1, phospho-p70S6K1 (Thr^{389}), phospho-STAT3 (Tyr^{705}), mTOR, phospho-mTOR (Ser^{2448}), 4E-BP1, phospho-4E-BP1 ($Thr^{37/46}$), eIF4E, phospho-eIF4E (Ser^{209}), phospho-CDC2 (Thr^{161}), CDC25C, phospho-CDC25C (Ser^{216}), Chk1, phospho-Chk1 (Ser^{345}), phospho-Chk2 (Thr^{168}), caspase-3, caspase-8, caspase-9, cleaved caspase-3, cleaved caspase-8, and LC3B were purchased from Cell Signaling Technology (Danvers, MA, USA). Antibodies for ERK 1/2, phospho-ERK 1/2 (Thr^{202}/Tyr^{204}), STAT3, CDC2, cyclin B1, cyclin A, Bcl-2, and Bcl-xL were purchased from Santa Cruz Biotechnology (Santa Cruz, CA, USA). Antibodies for VHL, PARP, cleaved PARP, and Bim were purchased from BD Pharmingen™ (BD Biosciences, San Jose, CA, USA). Hsp90 antibody was purchased from Stressgen Bioreagents (Ann Arbor, MI, USA).

3.2. Cell Culture

Human colorectal cancer cells (HCT116), gastric cancer cells (SNU638), breast cancer cells (MDA-MB-231), and liver cancer cells (SK-HEP-1) were purchased from American Type Culture Collection (Manassas, VA, USA). HCT116 and SNU638 cells were maintained in RPMI1640 medium, while MDA-MB-231 and SK-HEP-1 cells were cultured in DMEM medium that was supplemented with 10% heat-inactivated fetal bovine serum (FBS), 100 units/mL penicillin, 100 μg/mL streptomycin, and 250 ng/mL amphotericin B, respectively. Cells were maintained at 37 °C in a humidified atmosphere with 5% CO_2.

3.3. Sulforhodamine B Assay

HCT116 cells (2×10^4 cells/mL) were seeded in 96-well plates with various concentrations of SA and incubated at 37 °C in a humidified atmosphere with 5% CO_2. After incubation, the cells were fixed with a 50% trichloroacetic acid (TCA) solution for 1 h, and cellular proteins were stained with 0.4% sulforhodamine B (SRB) in 1% acetic acid. The stained cells were dissolved in 10 mM Tris buffer (pH 10.0). The effect of SA on cell proliferation was calculated as a percentage relative to a solvent-treated control, and the IC_{50} values were evaluated using nonlinear regression analysis (percent survival *versus* concentration).

3.4. Flow Cytometry for Cell Cycle and Apoptosis Analysis

HCT116 cells (2×10^5 cells/mL) were plated in a 36-mm culture dish and incubated for 24 h. Fresh medium containing the indicated concentration of SA was added to culture dishes. Following a 24 or 48 h incubation, the cells were harvested (via trypsinization and centrifugation), rinsed twice with pre-cooled phosphate buffered saline (PBS), and prepared for apoptosis and cell cycle analysis.

For cell cycle analysis, 1 mL of pre-cooled 70% ethanol was added, and the cells were fixed overnight at −20 °C. Next, fixed cells were washed with PBS and incubated with a staining solution containing RNase A (50 μg/mL) and propidium iodide (PI) (50 μg/mL) in PBS for 30 min at room temperature. The cellular DNA content was analyzed with a FACSCalibur® flow cytometer (BD Biosciences, San Jose, CA, USA). At least 10,000 cells were used for each analysis, and the distribution of cells in each phase of the cell cycle was displayed using histograms.

For apoptosis analysis, HCT116 cells were treated with the test compound for 48 h. After incubation, the cells were collected and washed twice with PBS. The cells were stained with Annexin V-FITC and propidium iodide (PI) solution using an Annexin V-FITC apoptosis detection kit (BD Biosciences) according to the manufacturer's instructions. In brief, HCT116 cells were diluted to 1×10^6 cells/mL. A 100 μL aliquot of cell suspension was transferred into a 15 mL round-bottom polystyrene tube, and 5 μL of PI solution were added to the cell suspension, which was further incubated for 20 min at room temperature in the dark. Stained cells were diluted with binding buffer and immediately analyzed by flow cytometry.

3.5. RNA Isolation and Real-Time Reverse Transcript-Polymerase Chain Reaction (RT-PCR)

RT-PCR was used to determine the gene expression of HIF-1α in HCT116 cells. Briefly, HCT116 cells (2×10^5 cells/mL) were cultured in 36-mm dishes for 24 h. The cells were then treated with various indicated concentrations of SA for an additional 8 h, with or without $CoCl_2$. Total cellular RNA was extracted with TRIzol reagent according to the manufacturer's instructions. The total RNA (1 μg) that was isolated from the cells was used for reverse transcription reaction with Reverse Transcription Reagents. The cDNA was reverse transcribed at 42 °C for 60 min with 0.5 μg of oligo $(dT)_{15}$ in a reaction volume of 20 μL using the reverse transcription system (Promega, MI, USA). Specific gene primers were designed and custom synthesized by Bioneer Corporation (Daejeon, Korea); HIF-1α forward: 5′-GATAGCAAGACTTTCCTCAGTCG-3′, reverse: 5′-TGGCCTCATATCCCATCAATTC-3′ and GUSβ forward: 5′-CTACATCGATGATGACATCACCGTCAC-3′, reverse: 5′-TGCCCTTGACAGAGATCTGGTAA-3′. Real-time PCR was conducted using a MiniOpticon system (Bio-Rad, Hercules, CA, USA); each PCR amplification included 5 μL of reverse transcription product, iQ SYBR Green Supermix (Bio-Rad, Hercules, CA, USA), and primers in a total volume of 20 μL. The following standard thermo cycler conditions were employed: 95 °C for 20 s prior to the first cycle; 40 cycles of 95 °C for 20 s, 56 °C for 20 s, and 72 °C for 30 s; 95 °C for 1 min; and 55 °C for 1 min. The threshold cycle (C_T), indicating the fractional cycle number at which the amount of amplified target gene reached a fixed threshold for each well, was determined using the MJ Opticon Monitor software package (Bio-Rad, Hercules, CA, USA). Relative quantification, representing the change in gene expression in real-time quantitative PCR experiments between a sample-treated group and the untreated control group, was calculated by the comparative C_T method in accordance with previously described methods [32]. The data were analyzed by evaluating the expression $2^{-\Delta\Delta CT}$, where $\Delta\Delta C_T$ = (C_T of target gene − C_T of housekeeping gene) treated group − (C_T of target gene − C_T of housekeeping gene) untreated control group. For the treated samples, the evaluation of $2^{-\Delta\Delta CT}$ represents the fold change in gene expression relative to the untreated control, normalized to a housekeeping gene (GUSβ).

3.6. Western Blot Analysis

HCT116 cells (2×10^5 cells/mL) were placed in a 36-mm culture dish and incubated for 24 h. A variety of concentrations of SA were then added, with or without $CoCl_2$, and the cells were cultured for the indicated time points before being digested. The protein was extracted with lysis buffer, and the protein concentrations were determined using the bicinchoninic acid (BCA) method. A 40 μg protein sample was collected from each group, boiled for 10 min, loaded onto 10% SDS-PAGE gels, and then transferred to PVDF membranes with electroblotting. Membranes were blocked for 1 h with 5% fat-free milk at room temperature, rinsed with PBS, and incubated with diluted primary antibodies 1:1000 or 1:500 overnight at 4 °C. Then, the membranes were incubated with specific secondary antibodies (1:1000) for 2 h and rinsed with PBS. The expression of β-actin was used as an internal standard.

Proteins were detected with an enhanced chemiluminescence detection kit from GE Healthcare (Little Chalfont, UK) and an LAS-4000 Imager (Fuji Film Corp., Tokyo, Japan).

3.7. Statistical Analysis

The data are presented as the mean ± SD for the indicated number of independently performed experiments. Statistical significance ($p < 0.05$) was assessed by one way analysis of variance (ANOVA) coupled with Dunnett's *t*-test.

4. Conclusions

Salternamide A was identified for the first time as an inhibitor of HIF-1α accumulation under hypoxic conditions in cancer cells (Figure 6). The translational regulation of HIF-1α accumulation by SA was partly associated with the down-regulation of the axis of the PI3K/mTOR/STAT3 signaling pathways. The anti-proliferative activity of SA in HCT116 colorectal cancer cells was also associated with G2/M cell cycle arrest and apoptotic/autophagic cell deaths. Therefore, SA is a leading candidate for the development of anticancer agents, and these mechanisms will be a key therapeutic target for pharmacologic and therapeutic intervention in HIF-1α-driven tumor growth and cell death.

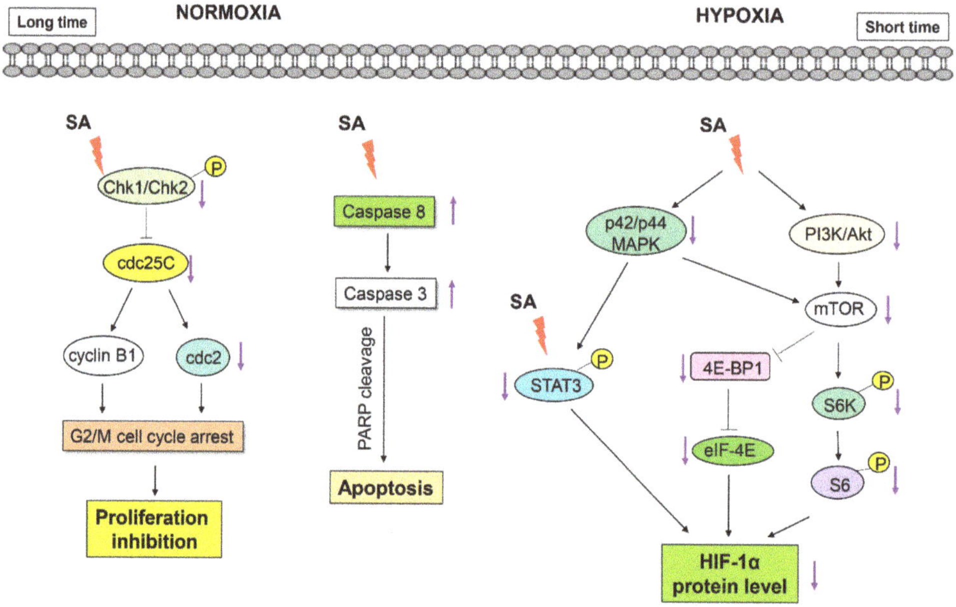

Figure 6. Proposed signaling pathways underlying the effects of SA on the suppression of HIF-1α and the induction of cell death in human colorectal cancer cells.

Acknowledgments: This work was supported by a National Research Foundation (NRF) grant funded by the Korean government (MEST) (NRF No. 2009-0083533) and a grant from the MarineBio Research Program of the NRF (NRF No. 2012-0006712).

Author Contributions: Duc-Hiep Bach and Sang Kook Lee conceived and designed the experiments; Duc-Hiep Bach performed the experiments; Seong-Hwan Kim and Dong-Chan Oh isolated the compound; Duc-Hiep Bach, Ji-Young Hong, Hyen Joo Park, and Sang Kook Lee analyzed the data; Duc-Hiep Bach, Ji-Young Hong, and Sang Kook Lee wrote the paper.

Conflicts of Interest: The authors declare no conflict of interest.

Abbreviations

HIF-1: hypoxia inducible factor-1; MG132: Z-Leu-Leu-Leu-al; Hsp90: heat-shock protein 90; VHL: Von Hippel-Lindau; Akt: oncogene from AKR mouse thymoma; PI3K: phosphoinositide 3-kinase; mTOR: mammalian target of rapamycin; p70S6K: p70 S6 kinase; 4E-BP1: initiation factor 4E-binding protein 1; RPS6: ribosomal protein S6; eIF4E: eukaryotic translation initiation factor 4E; VEGF: vascular endothelial growth factor; STAT3: signal transducer and activator of transcription-3; MAPK: mitogen-activated protein kinase; ERK: extracellular-signal-related kinase; LC3: light chain 3.

References

1. Feldser, D.; Agani, F.; Iyer, N.V.; Pak, B.; Ferreira, G.; Semenza, G.L. Reciprocal positive regulation of hypoxia-inducible factor 1alpha and insulin-like growth factor 2. *Cancer Res.* **1999**, *59*, 3915–3918. [PubMed]
2. Krishnamachary, B.; Berg-Dixon, S.; Kelly, B.; Agani, F.; Feldser, D.; Ferreira, G.; LaRusch, J.; Iyer, N.; Pak, B.; Taghavi, P.; *et al.* Regulation of colon carcinoma cell invasion by hypoxia-inducible factor 1. *Cancer Res.* **2003**, *63*, 1138–1143. [PubMed]
3. Pugh, C.W.; Ratcliffe, P.J. Regulation of angiogenesis by hypoxia: Role of the HIF system. *Nat. Med.* **2003**, *9*, 677–684. [CrossRef] [PubMed]
4. Semenza, G.L. Targeting HIF-1 for cancer therapy. *Nat. Rev. Cancer* **2003**, *3*, 721–732. [CrossRef] [PubMed]
5. Chen, C.; Pore, N.; Behrooz, A.; Ismail-Beigi, F.; Maity, A. Regulation of glut1 mRNA by hypoxia-inducible factor-1. Interaction between H-ras and hypoxia. *J. Biol. Chem.* **2001**, *276*, 9519–9525. [CrossRef] [PubMed]
6. Semenza, G.L.; Shimoda, L.A.; Prabhakar, N.R. Regulation of gene expression by HIF-1. *Novartis Found. Symp.* **2006**, *272*, 2–8. [PubMed]
7. Zhong, H.; de Marzo, A.M.; Laughner, E.; Lim, M.; Hilton, D.A.; Zagzag, D.; Buechler, P.; Isaacs, W.B.; Semenza, G.L.; Simons, J.W. Overexpression of hypoxia-inducible factor 1alpha in common human cancers and their metastases. *Cancer Res.* **1999**, *59*, 5830–5835. [PubMed]
8. Talks, K.L.; Turley, H.; Gatter, K.C.; Maxwell, P.H.; Pugh, C.W.; Ratcliffe, P.J.; Harris, A.L. The expression and distribution of the hypoxia-inducible factors HIF-1alpha and HIF-2alpha in normal human tissues, cancers, and tumor-associated macrophages. *Am. J. Pathol.* **2000**, *157*, 411–421. [CrossRef]
9. Semenza, G.L. HIF-1 and human disease: One highly involved factor. *Genes Dev.* **2000**, *14*, 1983–1991. [PubMed]
10. Zhong, H.; Chiles, K.; Feldser, D.; Laughner, E.; Hanrahan, C.; Georgescu, M.M.; Simons, J.W.; Semenza, G.L. Modulation of hypoxia-inducible factor 1alpha expression by the epidermal growth factor/phosphatidylinositol 3-kinase/PTEN/AKT/FRAP pathway in human prostate cancer cells: Implications for tumor angiogenesis and therapeutics. *Cancer Res.* **2000**, *60*, 1541–1545. [PubMed]
11. Richard, D.E.; Berra, E.; Gothie, E.; Roux, D.; Pouyssegur, J. p42/p44 mitogen-activated protein kinases phosphorylate hypoxia-inducible factor 1alpha (HIF-1alpha) and enhance the transcriptional activity of HIF-1. *J. Biol. Chem.* **1999**, *274*, 32631–32637. [CrossRef] [PubMed]
12. Sang, N.; Stiehl, D.P.; Bohensky, J.; Leshchinsky, I.; Srinivas, V.; Caro, J. MAPK signaling up-regulates the activity of hypoxia-inducible factors by its effects on p300. *J. Biol. Chem.* **2003**, *278*, 14013–14019. [CrossRef] [PubMed]
13. Yee Koh, M.; Spivak-Kroizman, T.R.; Powis, G. HIF-1 regulation: Not so easy come, easy go. *Trends Biochem. Sci.* **2008**, *33*, 526–534. [CrossRef] [PubMed]
14. Jung, J.E.; Lee, H.G.; Cho, I.H.; Chung, D.H.; Yoon, S.H.; Yang, Y.M.; Lee, J.W.; Choi, S.; Park, J.W.; Ye, S.K.; *et al.* STAT3 is a potential modulator of HIF-1-mediated VEGF expression in human renal carcinoma cells. *FASEB J.* **2005**, *19*, 1296–1298. [CrossRef] [PubMed]
15. Jung, J.E.; Kim, H.S.; Lee, C.S.; Shin, Y.J.; Kim, Y.N.; Kang, G.H.; Kim, T.Y.; Juhnn, Y.S.; Kim, S.J.; Park, J.W.; *et al.* STAT3 inhibits the degradation of HIF-1alpha by pVHL-mediated ubiquitination. *Exp. Mol. Med.* **2008**, *40*, 479–485. [CrossRef] [PubMed]
16. Kim, S.H.; Shin, Y.; Lee, S.H.; Oh, K.B.; Lee, S.K.; Shin, J.; Oh, D.C. Salternamides A-D from a Halophilic Streptomyces sp. Actinobacterium. *J. Nat. Prod.* **2015**, *78*, 836–843. [CrossRef] [PubMed]
17. Hansson, L.O.; Friedler, A.; Freund, S.; Rudiger, S.; Fersht, A.R. Two sequence motifs from HIF-1alpha bind to the DNA-binding site of p53. *Proc. Natl. Acad. Sci. USA* **2002**, *99*, 10305–10309. [CrossRef] [PubMed]
18. Creighton-Gutteridge, M.; Cardellina, J.H., 2nd; Stephen, A.G.; Rapisarda, A.; Uranchimeg, B.; Hite, K.; Denny, W.A.; Shoemaker, R.H.; Melillo, G. Cell type-specific, topoisomerase II-dependent inhibition of

hypoxia-inducible factor-1alpha protein accumulation by NSC 644221. *Clin. Cancer Res.* **2007**, *13*, 1010–1018. [CrossRef] [PubMed]

19. Liu, Y.V.; Baek, J.H.; Zhang, H.; Diez, R.; Cole, R.N.; Semenza, G.L. RACK1 competes with HSP90 for binding to HIF-1alpha and is required for O(2)-independent and HSP90 inhibitor-induced degradation of HIF-1alpha. *Mol. Cell* **2007**, *25*, 207–217. [CrossRef] [PubMed]
20. Zundel, W.; Schindler, C.; Haas-Kogan, D.; Koong, A.; Kaper, F.; Chen, E.; Gottschalk, A.R.; Ryan, H.E.; Johnson, R.S.; Jefferson, A.B.; *et al.* Loss of *PTEN* facilitates HIF-1-mediated gene expression. *Genes Dev.* **2000**, *14*, 391–396. [PubMed]
21. Noman, M.Z.; Buart, S.; van Pelt, J.; Richon, C.; Hasmim, M.; Leleu, N.; Suchorska, W.M.; Jalil, A.; Lecluse, Y.; el Hage, F.; *et al.* The cooperative induction of hypoxia-inducible factor-1 alpha and STAT3 during hypoxia induced an impairment of tumor susceptibility to CTL-mediated cell lysis. *J. Immunol.* **2009**, *182*, 3510–3521. [CrossRef] [PubMed]
22. Pawlus, M.R.; Wang, L.; Hu, C.J. STAT3 and HIF1alpha cooperatively activate HIF1 target genes in MDA-MB-231 and RCC4 cells. *Oncogene* **2014**, *33*, 1670–1679. [CrossRef] [PubMed]
23. Shrivastava, A.; Kuzontkoski, P.M.; Groopman, J.E.; Prasad, A. Cannabidiol induces programmed cell death in breast cancer cells by coordinating the cross-talk between apoptosis and autophagy. *Mol. Cancer Ther.* **2011**, *10*, 1161–1172. [CrossRef] [PubMed]
24. Mack, F.A.; Rathmell, W.K.; Arsham, A.M.; Gnarra, J.; Keith, B.; Simon, M.C. Loss of pVHL is sufficient to cause HIF dysregulation in primary cells but does not promote tumor growth. *Cancer Cell* **2003**, *3*, 75–88. [CrossRef]
25. Maranchie, J.K.; Vasselli, J.R.; Riss, J.; Bonifacino, J.S.; Linehan, W.M.; Klausner, R.D. The contribution of VHL substrate binding and HIF1-alpha to the phenotype of VHL loss in renal cell carcinoma. *Cancer Cell* **2002**, *1*, 247–255. [CrossRef]
26. Van den Beucken, T.; Koritzinsky, M.; Wouters, B.G. Translational control of gene expression during hypoxia. *Cancer Biol. Ther.* **2006**, *5*, 749–755. [CrossRef] [PubMed]
27. Niu, G.; Briggs, J.; Deng, J.; Ma, Y.; Lee, H.; Kortylewski, M.; Kujawski, M.; Kay, H.; Cress, W.D.; Jove, R.; *et al.* Signal transducer and activator of transcription 3 is required for hypoxia-inducible factor-1alpha RNA expression in both tumor cells and tumor-associated myeloid cells. *Mol. Cancer Res.* **2008**, *6*, 1099–1105. [CrossRef] [PubMed]
28. Pawlus, M.R.; Wang, L.; Murakami, A.; Dai, G.; Hu, C.J. STAT3 or USF2 contributes to HIF target gene specificity. *PLoS ONE* **2013**, *8*, e72358. [CrossRef] [PubMed]
29. Huang, W.W.; Ko, S.W.; Tsai, H.Y.; Chung, J.G.; Chiang, J.H.; Chen, K.T.; Chen, Y.C.; Chen, H.Y.; Chen, Y.F.; Yang, J.S. Cantharidin induces G2/M phase arrest and apoptosis in human colorectal cancer colo 205 cells through inhibition of CDK1 activity and caspase-dependent signaling pathways. *Int. J. Oncol.* **2011**, *38*, 1067–1073. [PubMed]
30. Doree, M.; Galas, S. The cyclin-dependent protein kinases and the control of cell division. *FASEB J.* **1994**, *8*, 1114–1121. [PubMed]
31. Peng, C.Y.; Graves, P.R.; Thoma, R.S.; Wu, Z.; Shaw, A.S.; Piwnica-Worms, H. Mitotic and G_2 checkpoint control: Regulation of 14-3-3 protein binding by phosphorylation of Cdc25C on serine-216. *Science* **1997**, *277*, 1501–1505. [CrossRef] [PubMed]
32. Dai, Y.; Grant, S. New insights into checkpoint kinase 1 in the DNA damage response signaling network. *Clin. Cancer Res.* **2010**, *16*, 376–383. [CrossRef] [PubMed]
33. Safarzadeh, E.; Sandoghchian Shotorbani, S.; Baradaran, B. Herbal medicine as inducers of apoptosis in cancer treatment. *Adv. Pharm. Bull.* **2014**, *4*, 421–427. [PubMed]
34. Dasari, S.; Tchounwou, P.B. Cisplatin in cancer therapy: Molecular mechanisms of action. *Eur. J. Pharmacol.* **2014**, *740*, 364–378. [CrossRef] [PubMed]

35. Gump, J.M.; Thorburn, A. Autophagy and apoptosis: What is the connection? *Trends Cell Biol.* **2011**, *21*, 387–392. [CrossRef] [PubMed]
36. Livesey, K.M.; Kang, R.; Vernon, P.; Buchser, W.; Loughran, P.; Watkins, S.C.; Zhang, L.; Manfredi, J.J.; Zeh, H.J., 3rd; Li, L.; *et al.* p53/HMGB1 complexes regulate autophagy and apoptosis. *Cancer Res.* **2012**, *72*, 1996–2005. [CrossRef] [PubMed]

marine drugs

Article

Synthesis and Antiplasmodial Evaluation of Analogues Based on the Tricyclic Core of Thiaplakortones A–D

Brett D. Schwartz [1], Mark J. Coster [1], Tina S. Skinner-Adams [1], Katherine T. Andrews [1], Jonathan M. White [2] and Rohan A. Davis [1,*]

[1] Eskitis Institute for Drug Discovery, Griffith University, Nathan, Qld 4111, Australia; b.schwartz@griffith.edu.au (B.D.S.); m.coster@griffith.edu.au (M.J.C.); t.skinner-adams@griffith.edu.au (T.S.S.); k.andrews@griffith.edu.au (K.T.A.)

[2] School of Chemistry and Bio21 Institute, University of Melbourne, Parkville, Vic 3052, Australia; whitejm@unimelb.edu.au

* Author to whom correspondence should be addressed; r.davis@griffith.edu.au; Tel.: +61-7-3735-6043; Fax: +61-7-3735-6001.

Academic Editor: Sylvia Urban
Received: 14 August 2015; Accepted: 7 September 2015; Published: 15 September 2015

Abstract: Six regioisomers associated with the tricyclic core of thiaplakortones A–D have been synthesized. Reaction of 1*H*-indole-4,7-dione and 1-tosyl-1*H*-indole-4,7-dione with 2-aminoethanesulfinic acid afforded a regioisomeric series, which was subsequently deprotected and oxidized to yield the tricyclic core scaffolds present in the thiaplakortones. All compounds were fully characterized using NMR and MS data. A single crystal X-ray structure was obtained on one of the *N*-tosyl derivatives. All compounds were screened for *in vitro* antiplasmodial activity against chloroquine-sensitive (3D7) and multidrug-resistant (Dd2) *Plasmodium falciparum* parasite lines. Several analogues displayed potent inhibition of *P. falciparum* growth (IC_{50} < 500 nM) but only moderate selectivity for *P. falciparum* versus human neonatal foreskin fibroblast cells.

Keywords: synthesis; thiaplakortone; regioisomer; tricyclic; natural product scaffold; X-ray; crystal; *Plasmodium falciparum*; antiplasmodial; cytotoxicity

1. Introduction

The marine natural products, thiaplakortones A–D (**1–4**), were first reported in 2013 as part of a Medicines for Malaria Venture sponsored research project that aimed to discover new antiplasmodial agents from nature (Figure 1) [1]. These unique thiazine-derived secondary metabolites were obtained from the organic extract from the Great Barrier Reef sponge *Plakortis lita*, and all were shown to inhibit the *in vitro* growth of *Plasmodium falciparum*. Thiaplakortone A (**1**) was the most active with *in vitro* IC_{50} values of 6.6 and 51 nM against multidrug-resistant (Dd2) and chloroquine-sensitive (3D7) *P. falciparum* lines, respectively [1]. Due to supply issues initially curtailing *in vivo* malaria studies, total syntheses of thiaplakortones A and B were undertaken and the first total synthesis of **1** and **2**, along with a series of mono- and di-methyl analogues (**5–7**) was subsequently reported and some preliminary structure-activity relationships (SAR) ascertained (Figure 1) [2]. While *in vivo* toxicity effects for several of the synthetic compounds indicated potential liabilities associated with this structure class, the limited number of analogues investigated made it difficult to assess their true potential as antiplasmodial leads [2]. In order to more thoroughly explore this compound class a larger analogue library based on the thiaplakortone A scaffold was recently undertaken and reported [3]. This 38-membered library consisted of a series of amide and urea analogues based on the thiaplakortone

A natural product scaffold. Several analogues showed potent *in vitro P. falciparum* growth inhibition (IC_{50} < 500 nM) and good selectivity for *P. falciparum* versus human neonatal foreskin fibroblast (NFF) cells (selectivity index >100) [3]. Furthermore, analogues **8** and **9** displayed good metabolic stability and solubility, and when administered subcutaneously to mice plasma concentrations remained >0.2 μM for 8 h. Analogues **8** and **9** were also well tolerated in mice after subcutaneous administration of 32 mg/kg twice daily for 4 d. In addition, using this dosing protocol blood stage *P. berghei* parasitemia was suppressed by 52% for **8** and 26% for **9**, relative to controls [3]. In order to further investigate the thiaplakortone core, we have recently undertaken synthetic studies that resulted in the removal of the ethylamine side-chain present in thiaplakortones A and B in order to determine the biological implications of the $-CH_2CH_2NH_2$ moiety. Herein we report the total synthesis of several side-chain truncated regioisomers associated with the tricyclic core of thiaplakortones A–D, along with their *in vitro* antiplasmodial activity and mammalian cell toxicity.

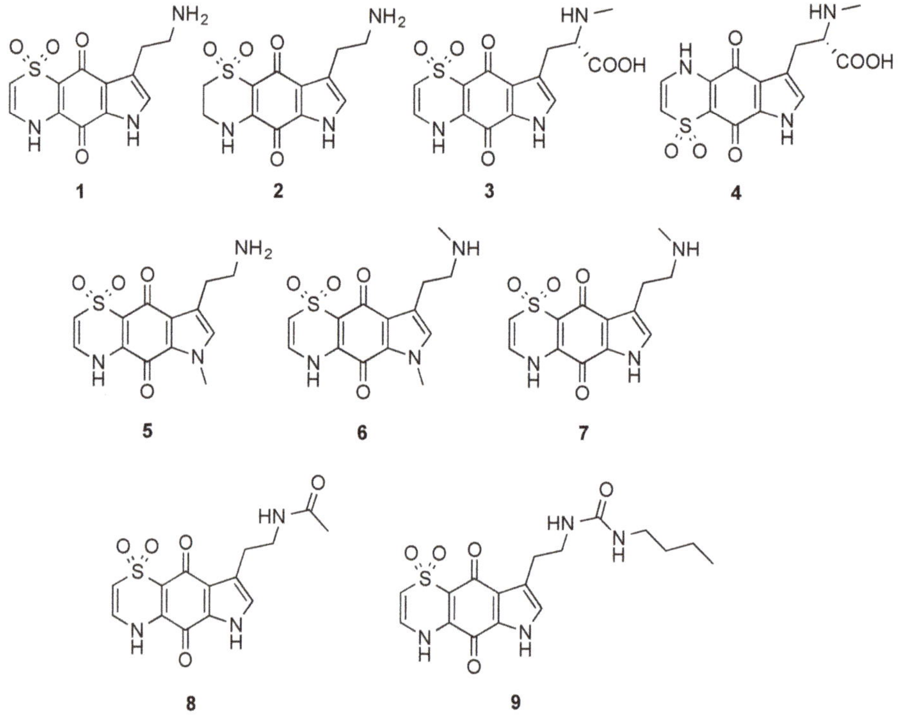

Figure 1. Chemical structures of the natural products thiaplakortones A–D (**1–4**) and some of the previously synthesized thiaplakortone A analogues (**5–9**).

2. Results and Discussion

2.1. Chemistry

The synthesis of the tricyclic core thiaplakortone isomers **11–16** commenced with the generation of 1-tosyl-1*H*-indole-4,7-dione (**10**), which was accessible via known procedures (Scheme 1) [4–6]. Condensation of **10** with 2-aminoethanesulfinic acid [2,7] furnished the regiomeric tricyclic systems **11** and **12** in an 11 to 1 ratio (Scheme 1). Separation of this mixture was not possible by silica flash chromatography however reversed-phase C_{18} HPLC (MeOH-H_2O-0.1%TFA) enabled separation of the two regioisomers. Confirmation of the chemical structures of **11** and **12** was supported following extensive 1D and 2D NMR data analysis.

Furthermore, a crystal suitable for X-ray analysis was obtained on the major regioisomer **11** (Figure 2) confirming the NMR-assigned structure and establishing the regiochemistry of subsequent compounds in the tricyclic series. Of note, compound **11** crystallized with two molecules in the asymmetric unit; the second molecule displayed disorder (*ca.* 13%) in the thiazine dioxide ring (see supplementary data).

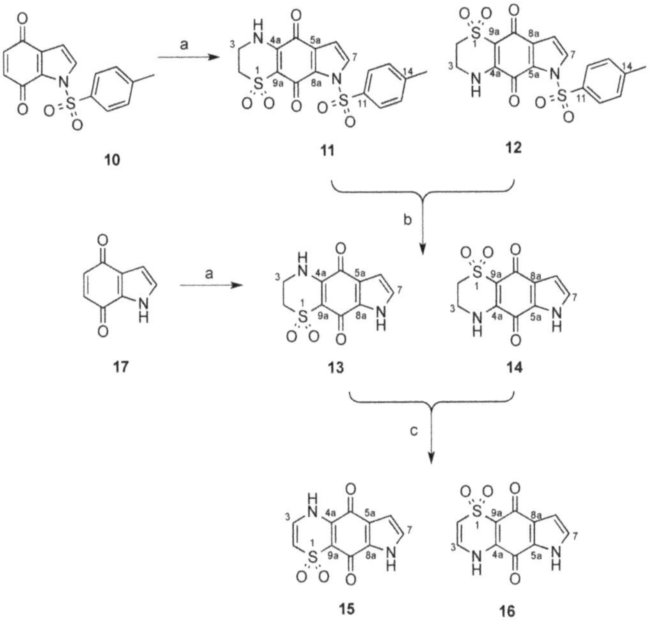

Scheme 1. Synthesis of compounds **11–16** in the thiaplakortone tricyclic series. (**a**) 2-aminoethanesulfinic acid, H_2O, MeCN; (**b**) $NaHCO_{3(aq)}$, MeOH, reflux 2.5 h; (**c**) $KOH_{(aq)}$, MeOH, O_2.

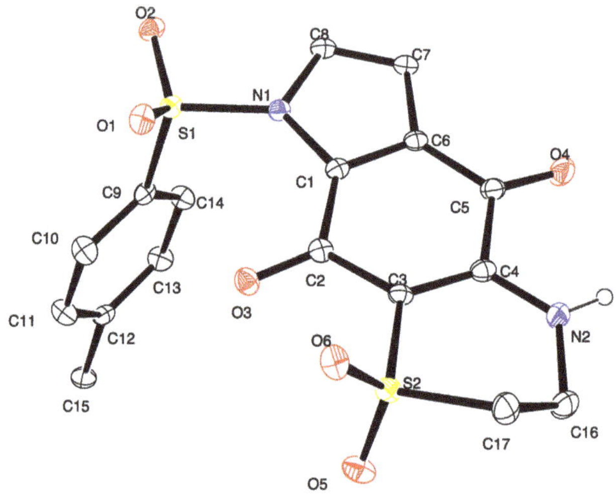

Figure 2. ORTEP diagram showing one independent molecule for compound **11**; ellipsoids are at the 30% probability level.

Subjection of the mixture of tosyl derivatives **11** and **12** to mild alkaline hydrolysis afforded a sufficient quantity of only compound **13** after purification by reversed-phase HPLC (MeOH-H_2O-0.1%TFA).

In an attempt to reverse the regioselectivity observed during the condensation of 2-aminoethanesulfinic acid with **10** and acquire suitable amounts of isomer **14**, the parent, non-tosyl protected system, 1*H*-indole-4,7-dione **17** was prepared according to literature procedures [5,8,9] and exposed to 2-aminoethanesulfinic acid. Gratifyingly, in this system, the opposite regioselectivity was observed and the respective tricyclic systems **13** and **14** were formed in a 1 to 3.3 ratio following analysis of the ^{1}H-NMR spectrum. Purification of this mixture by C_{18} HPLC (MeOH-H_2O-0.1%TFA) enabled **14** to be isolated in sufficient amounts for biological testing. Oxidation of the mixture of **13** and **14** by protocols previously reported [2] afforded a mixture that was subjected to C_{18} HPLC (MeOH-H_2O-0.1%TFA) and yielded the pure compounds **15** and **16**.

2.2. Biology and Structure-Activity Relationships

All compounds (**10–17**) were tested for *in vitro* antiplasmodial activity against chloroquine-sensitive (3D7) and multidrug-resistant (Dd2) *P. falciparum* parasite lines, and for mammalian toxicity using human neonatal foreskin fibroblast (NFF) cells. The simple indolequinones, **10** and **17**, were essentially inactive (Table 1), highlighting the importance of the 1,1-dioxo-thiazine subunit for antiplasmodial activity. The original thiaplakortone report [1] showed that unsaturation of the thiazine ring conferred enhanced antiplasmodial activity. This trend was also observed in the side-chain truncated compounds, with the unsaturated compounds, **15** and **16** displaying greater potency than their saturated counterparts, **13** and **14**, respectively. Specifically, exchanging the saturated system of **13** and **14** with the unsaturated motif present in **15** and **16** increased 3D7 activity by 23.9- and 27.3-fold, respectively; a similar SAR trend was also observed for this series towards the Dd2 line.

Table 1. Biological Data for Compounds **10–17**.

	Mean $IC_{50} \pm SD$ (nM)			
Compound	3D7 [a]	Dd2 [b]	NFF [c]	SI [d]
10	18,200 ± 2600	11,100 ± 4100	7600 ± 1200	0.4–0.7
11	546 ± 119	509 ± 309	1400 ± 700	2.6–2.8
12	834 ± 89	607 ± 158	19,000 ± 11,000	22.8–31.3
13	7500 ± 900	3800 ± 400	39,000 ± 4200	5.2–10.3
14	6900 ± 700	3700 ± 500	69,600 ± 5900	10.1–18.8
15	313 ± 84	129 ± 3.9	2800 ± 400	8.9–21.7
16	252 ± 35	127 ± 8.6	4600 ± 800	18.2–36.2
17	13,500 ± 6700	11,500 ± 6500	4700 ± 100	0.3–0.4
CQ [e]	7.8 ± 2.7	45 ± 10	36,500 ± 6000	811.1–4679.5

[a] 3D7 = *P. falciparum* chloroquine-sensitive line; [b] Dd2 = *P. falciparum* multidrug-resistant line; [c] NFF = neonatal foreskin fibroblast cells; [d] SI = selectivity index = NFF cell-line IC_{50}/*P. falciparum* IC_{50}; [e] CQ = chloroquine (positive control).

The regiochemistry of the thiazine moiety in the original thiaplakortone report was shown to have minimal influence on the overall antiplasmodial activity and selectivity [1]. Reversal of the thiazine orientation in thiaplakortones C (**3**) and D (**4**) only showed an antiplasmodial activity increase of 1.1-fold towards both the 3D7 and Dd2 lines. In a similar manner to the earlier report, the current studies showed minimal differences in parasite potency between the side-chain truncated regioisomeric pairs, **11** and **12**, **13** and **14**, and **15** and **16**. However, when comparing NFF toxicity of the regioisomers (**11** *vs.* **12**; **13** *vs.* **14**; **15** *vs.* **16**) a clear trend was observed, with the thiazine regiochemistry present in **12**, **14** and **16** conveying reduced cytotoxicity ranging from 1.6- to 13.6-fold. Furthermore, the reduction in toxicity improved the selectivity indices for analogues **12**, **14** and **16**.

Biological data for compounds **11** and **12** identified that *N*-tosylation of the pyrrole moiety is well tolerated and improves antiparasitic activity, even in the absence of thiazine unsaturation. It is interesting to note that, consistent with the thiaplakortone natural products [1], the most active side-chain truncated analogues, **15** and **16**, are more potent against the drug-resistant line (Dd2) than the chloroquine-sensitive line (3D7). While it is clear that the ethylamine side-chain present in thiaplakortones A and B translates to more potent and selective antiplasmodial agents, the current study shows that the tricyclic core motif present in **11–16** represents a minimum antiplasmodial pharmacophore for the thiaplakortone chemotype.

In order to assess the drug-like properties of compounds **10–17**, *in silico* physicochemical parameters (Table 2) were calculated using ChemAxon MarvinSketch software (with calculator plugins) (http://www.chemaxon.com) and the data compared to Lipinski's drug-like "Rule of Five" [10]. All compounds complied with Lipinski's rules (LogP < 5, HBA < 10, HBD < 5, MW < 500). In addition, all compounds had relatively low $LogD_{7.4}$ values (except compound **10**), and had appropriate polar surface area (PSA) values for membrane penetration.

Table 2. *In silico* physicochemical parameters for compounds **10–17** [a].

Compound	MW	LogP	HBA	HBD	PSA (Å^2)	$LogD_{7.4}$
10	301	1.5	4	0	82	1.9
11	406	−1.6	7	1	136	−0.2
12	406	−1.6	7	1	136	−0.2
13	252	−3.3	5	2	104	−1.6
14	252	−3.3	5	2	104	−1.6
15	250	−2.9	5	2	104	−1.5
16	250	−2.9	5	2	104	−1.5
17	147	−0.2	2	1	50	0.5

[a] *In silico* calculations performed using ChemAxon MarvinSketch software (with calculator plugins). MW = molecular weight (Da); HBA = H-bond acceptors; HBD = H-bond donors; PSA = polar surface area.

3. Experimental Section

3.1. General

Melting points were recorded on a capillary melting point apparatus and are uncorrected. Unless otherwise specified, ^1H and ^{13}C-NMR spectra were recorded at 30 °C in DMSO-d_6 on a Varian INOVA 500 or 600 NMR spectrometer. The ^1H- and ^{13}C-NMR chemical shifts were referenced to the solvent peak for DMSO-d_6 at δ_H 2.50 and δ_C 39.5. LRESIMS was obtained from LC-MS data generated using a Waters Alliance 2790 HPLC equipped with a Waters 996 photodiode array detector and an Alltech evaporative light scattering detector that was attached to a Water ZQ mass spectrometer. HRESIMS were recorded on a Bruker (Billerica, MA, USA) MicrOTof-Q spectrometer (Dionex UltiMate 3000 micro LC system, ESI mode). Analytical thin layer chromatography (TLC) was performed on aluminum-backed 0.2 mm thick silica gel 60 F_{254} plates as supplied by Merck (Frankfurt, Germany). Eluted plates were visualized using a 254 nm UV lamp and/or by treatment with a suitable dip followed by heating. These dips included phosphomolybdic acid:$Ce(SO_4)_2$:H_2SO_4 (conc.):H_2O (37.5 g:7.5 g:37.5 g:720 mL) or $KMnO_4$:K_2CO_3:5% NaOH aqueous solution:H_2O (3 g:20 g:5 mL:300 mL). Flash chromatographic separations were carried out following protocols defined by Still *et al.*, [11] with silica gel 60 (40–63 mm, supplied by GRACE, Baulkham Hills, NSW, Australia) or amino bonded silica gel (Davisil®) as the stationary phase and using the AR- or HPLC-grade solvents indicated. Semi-preparative HPLC work was performed using a Waters 600 pump and 966 PDA detector, a Gilson 715 liquid handler and a C_{18}-bonded silica Betasil 5 μm 143 Å column (21.2 mm × 150 mm). Alltech sample preparative C_{18}-bonded silica (35–75 μm, 150 Å) and an Alltech stainless steel guard cartridge (10 mm × 30 mm) were used for pre-adsorption and HPLC work. A Phenomenex C_{18}-bonded silica Luna 3 μm 100 Å (4.6 mm × 50 mm) column was used for LC-MS studies. All compounds were analyzed for purity using LC-MS and shown to be >95% pure, unless otherwise stated. Starting materials and reagents were available from the Sigma-Aldrich (St. Louis, MO, USA), Merck (Frankfurt, Germany), AK Scientific Inc. (Union City, CA, USA), Matrix Scientific Chemical (Columbia, SC, USA) and were used as supplied. MeOH and CH_2Cl_2 were dried using a glass contour solvent purification system that is based upon a technology originally described by Grubbs *et al.* [12]. Where necessary, reactions were performed under a nitrogen atmosphere and glassware was heated in an oven at 140 °C then dried under vacuum prior to use. Compounds for biological studies were placed under high vacuum (0.05 mmHg) for several hours before testing to remove trace, residual solvents.

3.2. Synthesis of N-Tosyl Regioisomers **11** and **12**

A solution of *N*-tosyl-1*H*-indole-4,7-dione (500 mg, 1.66 mmol) in MeCN (80 mL) was treated with a solution of 2-aminoethanesulfinic acid (236 mg, 2.16 mmol) in H_2O (50 mL) in one portion. The mixture was stirred for 20 h open to the atmosphere and then H_2O was removed by rotary evaporation and the resulting solid collected by vacuum filtration. The crystals were washed with H_2O (20 mL) then dried to afford a crude ~1:11 mixture of regioisomers **12** and **11**, respectively. This material (236 mg) was pre-adsorbed to C_{18}-bonded silica (1 g) overnight, then packed into a guard cartridge that was subsequently attached to a C_{18}-bonded silica semi-preparative HPLC column. Isocratic HPLC conditions of 90% H_2O (0.1% TFA)/10% MeOH (0.1% TFA) were employed for the first 10 min, then a linear gradient to MeOH (0.1% TFA) was run over 40 min, followed by isocratic conditions of MeOH (0.1% TFA) for a further 10 min, all at a flow rate of 9 mL/min. Sixty fractions (60 × 1 min) were collected by time from the start of the HPLC run. All UV active fractions were analyzed by ^1H-NMR spectroscopy and MS, and identical fractions were combined. This afforded **12** (7.6 mg, 1%, ^tR = 37.0–38.0 min) and **11** (69 mg, 10%, ^tR = 53.0–60.0 min). X-ray quality crystals of **11** were obtained through slow evaporation using a H_2O/MeOH (1:9) mix.

Compound **11**: Dull orange crystals (H_2O/MeOH); mp > 300 °C; ^1H-NMR (600 MHz, DMSO-d_6) δ_H 2.42 (3H, s, H-15), 3.27–3.29 (2H, m, H-2), 3.76–3.78 (2H, m, H-3), 6.83 (1H, d, *J* = 3.4 Hz, H-6), 7.50 (2H, d, *J* = 8.2 Hz, H-13), 7.90 (2H, d, *J* = 3.4 Hz, H-7), 8.01 (2H, d, *J* = 8.2 Hz, H-12), 9.01 (1H, br s,

H-4); ^{13}C-NMR (150 MHz, DMSO-d_6) δ_C 21.2 (C-15), 39.3 (C-3), 48.2 (C-2), 107.5 (C-6), 108.2 (C-9a), 126.7 (C-5a), 128.6 (2C, C-12), 129.3 (C-7), 129.8 (2C, C-13), 130.8 (C-8a), 133.5 (C-11), 146.2 (C-14), 146.6 (C-4a), 167.1 (C-9), 175.1 (C-5); (+)-LRESIMS m/z (rel. int.) 407 (100) $[M + H]^+$; (−)-LRESIMS m/z (rel. int.) 405 (100) $[M - H]^-$; (+)-HRESIMS m/z 429.0200 $[M + Na]^+$ (calcd for $C_{17}H_{14}N_2NaO_6S_2$, 429.0185).

Compound **12**: Bright orange amorphous solid; ^{1}H-NMR (600 MHz, DMSO-d_6) δ_H 2.41 (3H, s, H-15), 3.26–3.28 (2H, m, H-2), 3.75–3.77 (2H, m, H-3), 6.81 (1H, d, J = 3.2 Hz, H-8), 7.48 (2H, d, J = 8.4 Hz, H-13), 7.98 (2H, d, J = 8.4 Hz, H-12), 8.12 (2H, d, J = 3.2 Hz, H-7), 9.13 (1H, br s, H-4); ^{13}C-NMR (150 MHz, DMSO-d_6) δ_C 21.1 (C-15), 39.2 (C-3), 47.9 (C-2), 108.0 (C-9a), 108.8 (C-8), 125.9 (C-8a), 128.3 (2C, C-12), 130.0 (2C, C-13), 133.1 (C-11), 133.2 (C-7), 133.3 (C-5a), 146.4 (C-14), 147.4 (C-4a), 166.3 (C-5), 172.9 (C-9); (−)-LRESIMS m/z (rel. int.) 405 (100) $[M - H]^-$; (+)-LRESIMS m/z (rel. int.) 407 (100) $[M + H]^+$; (+)-HRESIMS m/z 429.0167 $[M + Na]^+$ (calcd for $C_{17}H_{14}N_2NaO_6S_2$, 429.0185).

3.3. Deprotection of the N-Tosyl Regioisomer Mixture to Yield 13

A 1:11 mixture of **12** and **11** (140 mg, 0.35 mmol) in a saturated solution of $NaHCO_3$ (5 mL) and MeOH (50 mL) was heated to reflux for 2.5 h. The mixture was acidified with HCl (32% aqueous) to pH 6 then concentrated and subjected to flash chromatography (silica, 1:10 v/v MeOH/CH_2Cl_2 elution) to afford a 1:26 mixture of compounds **14** and **13** (59 mg, 68%). This material (59 mg) was pre-adsorbed to C_{18}-bonded silica (1 g) overnight, then packed into a guard cartridge that was attached to a C_{18}-bonded silica semi-preparative HPLC column. Application of the same reversed-phase HPLC purification method described above (Section 3.2) afforded **13** (15 mg, 11%, ^{t}R = 23.0–24.0 min) as an orange powder.

Compound **13**: Orange amorphous solid; ^{1}H-NMR (500 MHz, DMSO-d_6) δ_H 3.31–3.33 (2H, m, H-2), 3.81–3.84 (2H, m, H-3), 6.57 (1H, d, J = 2.8 Hz, H-6), 7.13 (1H, d, J = 2.8 Hz, H-7), 9.05 (1H, brs, H-4), 12.76 (1H, brs, H-8); ^{13}C-NMR (125 MHz, DMSO-d_6) δ_C 39.4 (C-3), 48.2 (C-2), 107.5 (C-6), 120.7 (C-5a), 125.4 (C-7), 132.9 (C-8a), 148.2 (C-4a), 169.8 (C-9), 174.1 (C-5); (+)-LRESIMS m/z (rel. int.) 253 (100) $[M + H]^+$; (−)-LRESIMS m/z (rel. int.) 251 (100) $[M - H]^-$; (+)-HRESIMS m/z 275.0104 $[M + Na]^+$ (calcd for $C_{10}H_8N_2NaO_4S$, 275.0097).

3.4. Synthesis of Regioisomers 13 and 14

A solution of 1*H*-indole-4,7-dione (**10**, 504 mg, 3.4 mmol) in MeCN (160 mL) was treated with a solution of 2-aminoethanesulfinic acid (482 mg, 4.42 mmol) in H_2O (50 mL) in one portion and the mixture stirred for 20 h under an atmosphere of O_2. The MeCN and H_2O were removed by rotary evaporation to afford an orange solid, which was purified by flash chromatography (silica, 1:5 v/v MeOH/CH_2Cl_2 elution) to afford a 3.3:1 mixture of regioisomers **14** and **13**, respectively (307 mg, 36%). A portion of this material (40 mg) was pre-adsorbed to C_{18}-bonded silica (1 g) overnight, then packed into a guard cartridge that was attached to a C_{18}-bonded silica semi-preparative HPLC column. Isocratic HPLC conditions of 95% H_2O (0.1% TFA)/5% MeOH (0.1% TFA) were employed for the first 10 min, then a linear gradient to 50% H_2O (0.1% TFA)/50% MeOH (0.1% TFA) was run over 40 min, followed by a linear gradient to MeOH (0.1% TFA) in 1 min, then isocratic conditions of MeOH (0.1% TFA) for a further 9 min, all at a flow rate of 9 mL/min. Sixty fractions (60 × 1 min) were collected by time from the start of the HPLC run. All UV active fractions were analyzed by ^{1}H-NMR spectroscopy and MS, and identical fractions were combined. This yielded **14** (5.0 mg, 1%, ^{t}R = 25.0–27.0 min) as a bright orange powder.

Compound **14**: Bright orange amorphous solid; ^{1}H-NMR (500 MHz, DMSO-d_6) δ_H 3.28–3.33 (2H, m, H-2), 3.79–3.82 (2H, m, H-3), 6.53 (1H, d, J = 2.5 Hz, H-8), 7.40 (1H, d, J = 2.5 Hz, H-7), 8.89 (1H, br s, H-4), 12.81 (1H, br s, H-6); ^{13}C-NMR (125 MHz, DMSO-d_6) δ_C 39.3 (C-3), 48.4 (C-2), 108.4 (2C, C-9a, C-8), 127.2 (C-8a), 128.2 (C-5a), 130.1 (C-7), 147.5 (C-4a), 167.9 (C-5), 174.7 (C-9); (+)-LRESIMS m/z (rel. int.) 253 (100) $[M + H]^+$; (−)-LRESIMS m/z (rel. int.) 251 (100) $[M - H]^-$; (+)-HRESIMS m/z 275.0087 $[M + Na]^+$ (calcd for $C_{10}H_8N_2NaO_4S$, 275.0097).

3.5. Synthesis of Regioisomers **15** and **16**

A 3.3:1 regioisomeric mixture of **14** and **13** (90 mg, 0.36 mmol) from the synthesis described above (Section 3.4) in a solution of MeOH (10 mL) was treated with an aqueous KOH solution (6 mL, 12 M). The magnetically stirred reaction mixture was purged with O_2, and maintained at 60 °C under a balloon of O_2 for 4 h. The reaction mixture was cooled to 0 °C, carefully neutralized by the addition of an aqueous solution of HCl (1 M) and then the mixture was concentrated *in vacuo* to afford a residue that was subjected to flash chromatography through a small plug of silica (1:10 v/v MeOH/CH_2Cl_2 elution) and after concentration of the eluent *in vacuo*, the residue (40 mg) was pre-adsorbed to C_{18}-bonded silica (1 g) overnight, then packed into a guard cartridge that was attached to a C_{18}-bonded silica semi-preparative HPLC column. Application of same reversed-phase HPLC purification method described above (Section 3.4) resulted in the purification of compounds **16** (15 mg, 17%, ^{t}R = 28.0–30.0 min) and **15** (5 mg, 6%, ^{t}R = 32.0–34.0 min) as yellow and orange powders, respectively.

Compound **15**: Orange amorphous solid; ^{1}H-NMR (500 MHz, DMSO-d_6) δ_H 6.49 (1H, d, J = 8.8 Hz, H-2), 6.66 (1H, d, J = 2.8 Hz, H-6), 7.07 (1H, d, J = 8.8 Hz, H-3), 7.27 (1H, d, J = 2.8 Hz, H-7), 11.07 (1H, br s, H-4), 12.99 (1H, br s, H-8); ^{13}C-NMR (125 MHz, DMSO-d_6) δ_C 108.0 (C-6), 111.7 (C-2), 113.4 (C-9a), 121.8 (C-5a), 126.8 (C-7), 130.2 (C-3), 131.3 (C-8a), 140.5 (C-4a), 172.2 (C-9), 174.1 (C-5); (+)-LRESIMS m/z (rel. int.) 251 (100) $[M + H]^+$; (−)-LRESIMS m/z (rel. int.) 249 (100) $[M - H]^-$; (+)-HRESIMS m/z 272.9939 $[M + Na]^+$ (calcd for $C_{10}H_6N_2NaO_4S$, 272.9940).

Compound **16**: Yellow amorphous solid; ^{1}H NMR (500 MHz, DMSO-d_6) δ_H 6.42 (1H, d, J = 8.8 Hz, H-2), 6.60 (1H, d, J = 2.6 Hz, H-8), 7.04 (1H, d, J = 8.8 Hz, H-3), 7.43 (1H, d, J = 2.6 Hz, H-7), H-4 and H-6 not observed; ^{13}C-NMR (125 MHz, DMSO-d_6) δ_C 108.5 (C-8), 111.6 (C-2), 113.9 (C-9a), 126.9 (C-8a), 127.6 (C-5a), 129.8 (C-7), 130.1 (C-3), 140.2 (C-4a), 167.9 (C-5), 177.3 (C-9); (+)-LRESIMS m/z (rel. int.) 251 (100) $[M + H]^+$; (−)-LRESIMS m/z (rel. int.) 249 (100) $[M - H]^-$; (+)-HRESIMS m/z 272.9933 $[M + Na]^+$ (calcd for $C_{10}H_6N_2NaO_4S$, 272.9940).

3.6. X-ray Crystallography Studies on Compound **11**

Intensity data were collected with an Oxford Diffraction SuperNova CCD diffractometer using Cu-Kα radiation, the temperature during data collection was maintained at 100.0(1) using an Oxford Cryosystems cooling device. The structure was solved by direct methods and difference Fourier Synthesis [13]. Hydrogen atoms bound to the carbon atom were placed at their idealized positions using appropriate HFIX instructions in SHELXL, and included in subsequent refinement cycles. Hydrogen atoms attached to nitrogen were located from difference Fourier maps and refined freely with isotropic displacement parameters. Thermal ellipsoid plots were generated using the program ORTEP-3 [14] integrated within the WINGX suite of programs [15]. Full details of the data collection and refinement and tables of atomic coordinates, bond lengths and angles, and torsion angles have been deposited with the Cambridge Crystallographic Data Centre (CCDC 1416796). Copies can be obtained free of charge on application at the following address: http://www.ccdc.cam.ac.uk.

Crystal data for compound **11**: $C_{17}H_{14}N_2O_6S_2$, M = 406.42, T = 100.0(2) K, λ = 1.5418 Å, Triclinic, space group $P2_1/c$, a = 11.6802(7), b = 28.0975(14), c = 10.3047(6) Å, β = 91.539(5)° V = 3380.6(3) Å^3, Z = 8, Z' = 2, D_c = 1.597 Mg·M^{-3}, μ = 3.230 mm^{-1}, $F(000)$ = 1680, crystal size 0.49 mm × 0.38 mm × 0.31 mm. θ_{max} = 67.6°, 10,831 reflections measured, 5907 independent reflections (R_{int} = 0.051) the final R = 0.0559 [$I > 2\sigma(I)$, 5134 data] and $wR(F^2)$ = 0.1577 (all data) GOOF = 1.027.

3.7. P. Falciparum Growth Inhibition Assay

P. falciparum growth inhibition assays were carried out using an isotopic microtest, as previously described [16]. Briefly, *in vitro* cultured *P. falciparum* infected erythrocytes (1.0% parasitemia and 1.0% hematocrit) were seeded into triplicate wells of 96 well tissue culture plates containing vehicle control (DMSO), positive control [chloroquine (Sigma-Aldrich, St. Louis, MO, USA), catalogue #C6628, >98%] or test compounds and incubated under standard *P. falciparum* culture conditions with 0.5

μCi [^{3}H]-hypoxanthine. The final concentration of DMSO vehicle was <0.5% in all assay wells (non-toxic). After 48 h cells were harvested onto 1450 MicroBeta filter mats (PerkinElmer, Waltham, Massachusetts, USA) and [^{3}H] incorporation determined using a 1450 MicroBeta liquid scintillation counter. Percentage inhibition of growth compared to matched DMSO controls was determined and IC_{50} values were calculated using linear interpolation of inhibition curves [17]. The mean IC_{50} or % inhibition (±SD) was calculated for three independent experiments, each carried out in triplicate.

4. Conclusions

In summary, six analogues associated with the tricyclic core of thiaplakortones were synthesized from readily accessible and known 1*H*-indole-4,7-dione derivatives, and isolated in low to moderate yields. Regiochemistry was moderated by substitution of the indole nitrogen. All compounds were tested for *in vitro* antiplasmodial activity towards two *P. falciparum* parasite lines (3D7 and Dd2). Compound **16** showed the best antiparasitic activity with IC_{50} values of 252 and 127 nM towards 3D7 and Dd2 lines, respectively. The moderate toxicity (IC_{50} 4600 nM) of compound **16** towards NFF cells equates to a selectivity index of 18.2–36.2. These studies have identified that while the ethylamine side-chain present in the marine natural products, thiaplakortones A and B, translates to more potent and selective antiplasmodial compounds, this functionality is by no means essential for activity. Furthermore, the truncated thiaplakortone molecules (**11–16**) synthesized during this work has allowed delineation of a minimum antiplasmodial pharmacophore for the thiaplakortone chemotype.

Acknowledgments: We thank the National Health and Medical Research Council (NHMRC) for financial support towards this research through a project grant (APP1024314). R.A.D. and K.T.A. acknowledge the Australian Research Council (ARC) for an ARC Linkage Grant (LP120200339) and an ARC Future Fellowship, respectively. We also thank the ARC for support toward NMR and MS equipment (Grant LE0668477 and LE0237908). G. MacFarlane (University of Queensland) and W. Loa (Griffith University) are acknowledged for HRESIMS measurements. We also acknowledge the Australian Red Cross Blood Service for the provision of human blood and sera.

Author Contributions: B.D.S. designed and conducted all synthetic experiments and analyzed the results. T.S.S. and K.T.A. designed and performed all the biological experiments, and contributed to data interpretation. M.J.C. assisted with synthetic experimental design, and SAR data analysis. J.M.W. obtained the X-ray diffraction data for compound **11**, and solved the crystal structure. R.A.D. was the project leader overseeing the design of the experiments, analysis of the results and the identification and characterization of all compounds. All authors contributed to manuscript preparation.

Conflicts of Interest: The authors declare no conflict of interest.

References

1. Davis, R.A.; Duffy, S.; Fletcher, S.; Avery, V.M.; Quinn, R.J. Thiaplakortones A-D: Antimalarial Thiazine Alkaloids from the Australian Marine Sponge *Plakortis lita*. *J. Org. Chem.* **2013**, *78*, 9608–9613. [CrossRef] [PubMed]
2. Pouwer, R.H.; Deydier, S.M.; Le, P.V.; Schwartz, B.D.; Franken, N.C.; Davis, R.A.; Coster, M.J.; Charman, S.A.; Edstein, M.D.; Skinner-Adams, T.S.; *et al.* Total Synthesis of Thiaplakortone A: Derivatives as Metabolically Stable Leads for the Treatment of Malaria. *ACS Med. Chem. Lett.* **2013**, *5*, 178–182. [CrossRef] [PubMed]
3. Schwartz, B.; Skinner-Adams, T.; Andrews, K.T.; Coster, M.; Edstein, M.; MacKenzie, D.; Charman, S.; Koltun, M.; Blundell, S.; Campbell, A.; *et al.* Synthesis and antimalarial evaluation of amide and urea derivatives based on the thiaplakortone A natural product scaffold. *Org. Biomol. Chem.* **2015**, *13*, 1558–1570. [CrossRef] [PubMed]
4. Hollis Showalter, H.D.; Pohlmann, G. An Improved Synthesis of 4,7-Dimethoxy-1*H*-Indole. *Org. Prep. Proc. Int.* **1992**, *24*, 484–488. [CrossRef]
5. Jackson, Y.A.; Billimoria, A.D.; Sadanandan, E.V.; Cava, M.P. Regioselective Amination of Indole-4,7-quinones. *J. Org. Chem.* **1995**, *60*, 3543–3545. [CrossRef]
6. Rajeswari, S.; Drost, K.J.; Cava, M.P. A convenient reductive cyclization of β,2-dinitrostyrenes to indoles. *Heterocycles* **1989**, *29*, 415.
7. Schmitz, F.J.; Bloor, S.J. Xesto- and halenaquinone derivatives from a sponge, *Adocia* sp., from Truk lagoon. *J. Org. Chem.* **1988**, *53*, 3922–3925. [CrossRef]

8. Cherif, M.; Cotelle, P.; Catteau, J.P. General synthesis of 2,3-substituted 5-membered heterocyclic quinones. *Heterocycles* **1992**, *34*, 1749–1758.
9. Kitahara, Y.; Nakahara, S.; Numata, R.; Kubo, A. Synthesis of 4,7-Indolequinones. The Oxidative Demethylation of 4,7-Dimethoxyindoles with Ceric Ammonium Nitrate. *Chem. Pharm. Bull.* **1985**, *33*, 2122–2128. [CrossRef]
10. Lipinski, C.A.; Lombardo, F.; Dominy, B.W.; Feeney, P.J. Experimental and computational approaches to estimate solubility and permeability in drug discovery and development settings. *Adv. Drug Deliv. Rev.* **2001**, *46*, 3–26. [CrossRef]
11. Still, W.C.; Kahn, M.; Mitra, A. Rapid chromatographic technique for preparative separations with moderate resolution. *J. Org. Chem.* **1978**, *43*, 2923–2925. [CrossRef]
12. Pangborn, A.B.; Giardello, M.A.; Grubbs, R.H.; Rosen, R.K.; Timmers, F.J. Safe and Convenient Procedure for Solvent Purification. *Organometallics* **1996**, *15*, 1518–1520. [CrossRef]
13. Sheldrick, G.M. A short history of SHELX. *Acta Cryst.* **2008**, *A64*, 112–122. [CrossRef] [PubMed]
14. Farrugia, L.J. ORTEP-3 for windows—A version of ORTEP-III with a graphical user interface (GUI). *J. Appl. Cryst.* **1997**, *30*, 565. [CrossRef]
15. Farrugia, L.J. WinGX suite for small-molecule single-crystal crystallography. *J. Appl. Cryst.* **1999**, *32*, 837–838. [CrossRef]
16. Skinner, T.S.; Manning, L.S.; Johnston, W.A.; Davis, T.M. E. *In vitro* stage-specific sensitivity of *Plasmodium falciparum* to quinine and artemisinin drugs. *Int. J. Parasitol.* **1996**, *26*, 519–525. [CrossRef]
17. Huber, W.; Koella, J.C. A comparison of three methods of estimating EC_{50} in studies of drug resistance of malaria parasites. *Acta Trop.* **1993**, *55*, 257–261. [CrossRef]

marine drugs

MDPI

Article

Structure-Activity Relationships of the Bioactive Thiazinoquinone Marine Natural Products Thiaplidiaquinones A and B

Jacquie L. Harper [1], Iman M. Khalil [2], Lisa Shaw [1,†], Marie-Lise Bourguet-Kondracki [3], Joëlle Dubois [4], Alexis Valentin [5], David Barker [2] and Brent R. Copp [2,*]

[1] Malaghan Institute of Medical Research, PO Box 7060 Wellington South, New Zealand; jharper@malaghan.org.nz (J.L.H); l.shaw@centenary.org.au (L.S.)

[2] School of Chemical Sciences, University of Auckland, Private Bag 92019, 1142 Auckland, New Zealand; ikha019@aucklanduni.ac.nz (I.M.K.); d.barker@auckland.ac.nz (D.B.)

[3] Laboratoire Molécules de Communication et Adaptation des Micro-organismes, UMR 7245 CNRS, Muséum National d'Histoire Naturelle, 57 rue Cuvier (C.P. 54), 75005 Paris, France; bourguet@mnhn.fr

[4] Institut de Chimie des Substances Naturelles, CNRS UPR 2301, Centre de Recherche de Gif, Avenue de la Terrasse, 91198 Gif sur Yvette Cedex, France; joelle.dubois@icsn.cnrs-gif.fr

[5] Université Paul Sabatier, PHARMA-DEV, UMR 152 IRD-UPS, Université de Toulouse, 118 Route de Narbonne, F-31062 Toulouse cedex 9, France; alexis.valentin@univ-tlse3.fr

* Author to whom correspondence should be addressed; b.copp@auckland.ac.nz; Tel.: +64-9-373-7599; Fax: +64-9-373-7422.

† Present Address: Centenary Institute, Royal Prince Alfred Hospital, Missenden Rd, Camperdown, NSW 2050, Australia.

Academic Editor: Sylvia Urban

Received: 15 July 2015; Accepted: 4 August 2015; Published: 10 August 2015

Abstract: In an effort to more accurately define the mechanism of cell death and to establish structure-activity relationship requirements for the marine meroterpenoid alkaloids thiaplidiaquinones A and B, we have evaluated not only the natural products but also dioxothiazine regioisomers and two precursor quinones in a range of bioassays. While the natural products were found to be weak inducers of ROS in Jurkat cells, the dioxothiazine regioisomer of thiaplidiaquinone A and a synthetic precursor to thiaplidiaquinone B were found to be moderately potent inducers. Intriguingly, and in contrast to previous reports, the mechanism of Jurkat cell death (necrosis *vs.* apoptosis) was found to be dependent upon the positioning of one of the geranyl sidechains in the compounds with thiaplidiaquinone A and its dioxothiazine regioisomer causing death dominantly by necrosis, while thiaplidiaquinone B and its dioxothiazine isomer caused cell death *via* apoptosis. The dioxothiazine regioisomer of thiaplidiaquinone A exhibited more potent *in vitro* antiproliferative activity against human tumor cells, with NCI sub-panel selectivity towards melanoma cell lines. The non-natural dioxothiazine regioisomers were also more active in antiplasmodial and anti-farnesyltransferase assays than their natural product counterparts. The results highlight the important role that natural product total synthesis can play in not only helping understand the structural basis of biological activity of natural products, but also the discovery of new bioactive scaffolds.

Keywords: thiaplidiaquinone; *Aplidium*; ascidian; thiazinoquinone; apoptosis; Jurkat; cytotoxicity; malaria; farnesyltransferase

1. Introduction

The structures of marine natural products continue to provide not only targets for total synthesis but also new templates for biological evaluation. Ascidians of the genus *Aplidium* are a notable source of structurally complex natural products, including meroterpenoids, many of which exhibit potentially useful biological properties [1]. In addition to our own discoveries of rossinone B (potent cytotoxin) from an Antarctic *Aplidium* sp. [2] and scabellone B (antimalarial) from a New Zealand collection of *Aplidium scabellum* [3], Fattorusso's group reported the structures of thiaplidiaquinones A (**1**) and B (**2**), two thiazine-meroterpenoids, from Mediterranean specimens of *Aplidium conicum* (Figure 1) [4]. Both **1** and **2** exhibited cytotoxicity towards the human leukemia T cell line Jurkat with IC_{50} ~3 μM with propidium iodide staining and flow cytometry data indicating that the natural products increased the frequency of subdiploid (apoptotic) cells caused by a rapid overproduction of intracellular reactive oxygen species (ROS) which in-turn led to a collapse of the mitochondrial transmembrane potential.

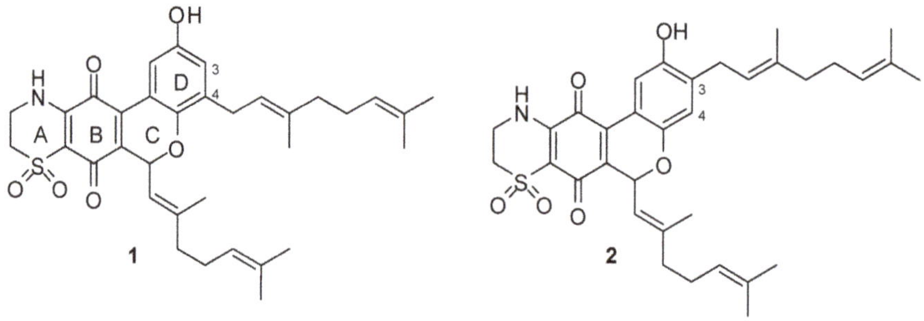

Figure 1. Structures of natural products thiaplidiaquinone A (**1**) and thiaplidiaquinone B (**2**).

The interesting structures of thiaplidiaquinones A and B and their associated biological activities piqued the interest of ourselves and others, leading to reported biomimetic syntheses of **1** and **2** [5,6]. In addition to natural products **1** and **2**, our synthesis also led to the corresponding dioxothiazine isomers **3** and **4**. To investigate elements of the structural basis of ROS generation and Jurkat cell line cytotoxicity reported for the isolated natural products **1** and **2** [4], we have evaluated **1–6** in a similar set of assays and have also included more comprehensive evaluation for antitumor activity at the National Cancer Institute (USA) as well as for antimalarial and anti-farnesyltransferase activities.

2. Results and Discussion

2.1. Chemistry

The biomimetic syntheses of thiaplidiaquinones A and B and their corresponding thiazine regioisomers **3** and **4** *via* precursor quinones **5** and **6** (Figure 2) have been reported elsewhere [5].

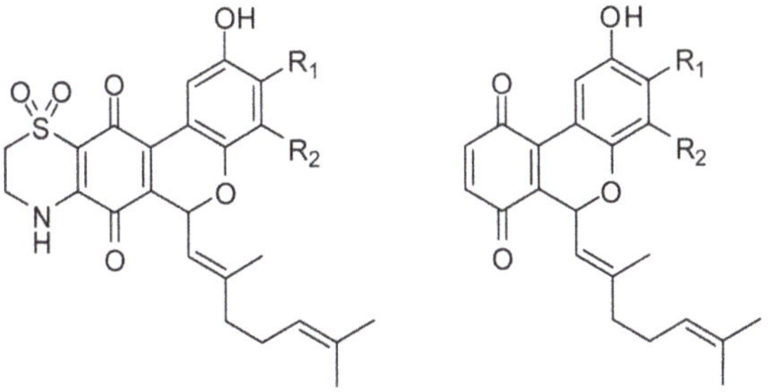

Figure 2. Structures of thiazine regioisomers **3** and **4** and precursor quinones **5** and **6**.

2.2. Biology

2.2.1. Inhibition of ROS Generation

It was originally reported that thiaplidiaquinones A and B displayed a strong accumulation of intracellular ROS in Jurkat cells, 97% of cells for **1** and 93% for **2**, relative to untreated cells [4]. In the present study, the presence of ROS in Jurkat cells was determined using dihydrorhodamine 123 (DHR123), a cell permeable probe that becomes fluorescent when oxidized to rhodamine 123 in the presence of ROS [7]. Once the cells were loaded with DHR123, they were then treated with test compounds at a range of concentrations, and the mean fluorescent intensity determined by flow cytometry. In Figure 3 it is shown that even at a top test concentration of 100 μM, natural products **1** and **2** exhibited only modest levels of accumulation of intracellular ROS, particularly in comparison to precursor quinones **5** and **6** and the dioxothiazine regioisomer of thiaplidiaquinone A **3**. Of the four dioxothiazine-containing compounds (**1–4**), **3** was clearly the most potent generator of intracellular ROS in this assay.

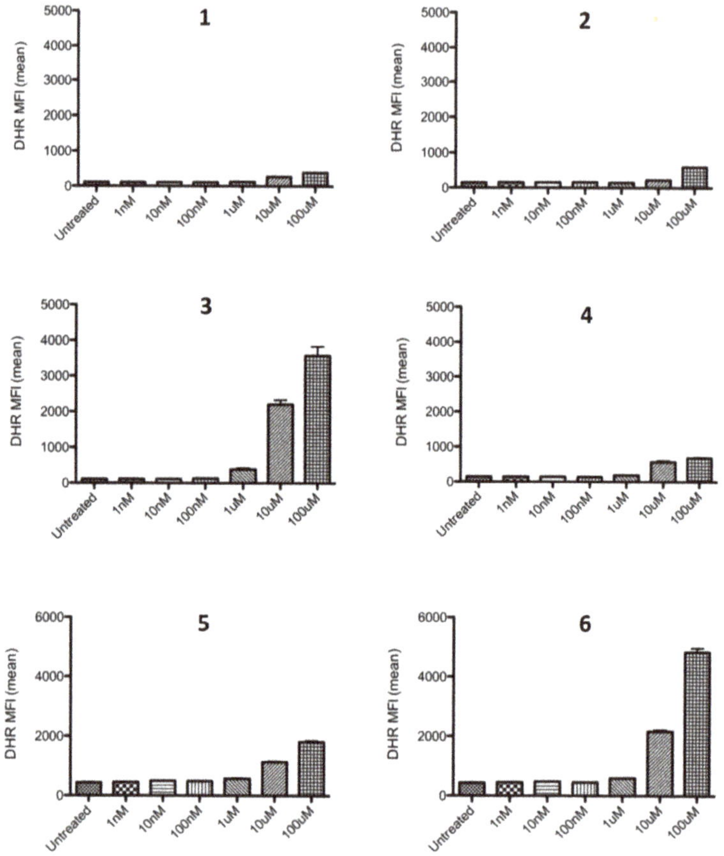

Figure 3. Comparison of DHR fluorescence by Jurkat cells treated with **1–6**.

2.2.2. Apoptosis *vs.* Necrosis in Jurkat Cells

It was reported previously that natural products **1** and **2** exhibited similar levels of cytotoxicity towards Jurkat cells with IC_{50} ~3 μM using a standard cell viability assay [4]. In addition, by using propidium iodide (PI) as a probe, from the observation of treated cells having a significant loss of nuclear DNA in combination with ROS production it was concluded that both **1** and **2** were inducing apoptosis. However, as this approach looked at the average cell population it does not provide the opportunity to clearly differentiate between apoptosing and necrosing cell subpopulations. In our hands, natural products **1** and **2**, and regioisomers **3** and **4**, exhibited significantly less potent cytotoxicity towards Jurkat cells, with toxicity only apparent at concentrations close to 100 μM. For our assessment of the mechanism of cell death, we used the combination of Annexin V-FITC and PI stains to allow us to evaluate the ability of test compounds **1–6** to induce apoptosis or necrosis (or both) in Jurkat cells. After 24 h treatment in the presence of 100 μM of each test compound, cells were analyzed by flow cytometry to identify live (AnV^-/PI^-), apoptosing (AnV^+/PI^-), necrotic (AnV^-/PI^+) and late apoptotic (AnV^+/PI^+) cells.

As shown in Figure 4, natural products thiaplidiaquinone A (**1**) and B (**2**) exhibited quite different profiles, with **1** inducing both necrosis (PI^+/AV^-) and apoptosis (PI^-/AV^+) and **2** causing cell death almost exclusively *via* apoptosis. A similar profile was observed for the dioxothiazine regioisomers **3** and **4**, with an even clearer distinction between cell death by necrosis for **3**, while cell death induced by **4** was dominantly *via* apoptosis. These results identify that placement of the geranyl side chain in ring-D of the molecule specifically dictates the mechanism of cell death (**1**/**3** *vs.* **2**/**4**) with a geranyl chain at the C-3 position resulting in death by apoptosis in comparison to a geranyl chain at the C-4 position which results in necrotic cell death. In direct contrast to the dioxothiazine-containing compounds, the profiles of both precursor quinones **5** and **6** were dominated by late stage apoptosis (PI^+/AV^+). From the observations made, it is evident that the presence of the dioxothiazine ring modulates the activity of the compounds (*i.e.*, **1**–**4** *vs.* **5**/**6**) whereas the placement of one of the geranyl side chains in the structure specifically dictates the mechanism of cell death (**1**/**3** *vs.* **2**/**4**). It should be noted that the induction of ROS did not clearly correlate with either apoptotic or necrotic cell death indicating that ROS production appears to be a poor indicator of the route of cell death for the current test compounds. This is not unexpected as necrosis is also linked to ROS production [8,9], thereby confounding the use of ROS as an indicator of the route of cell death.

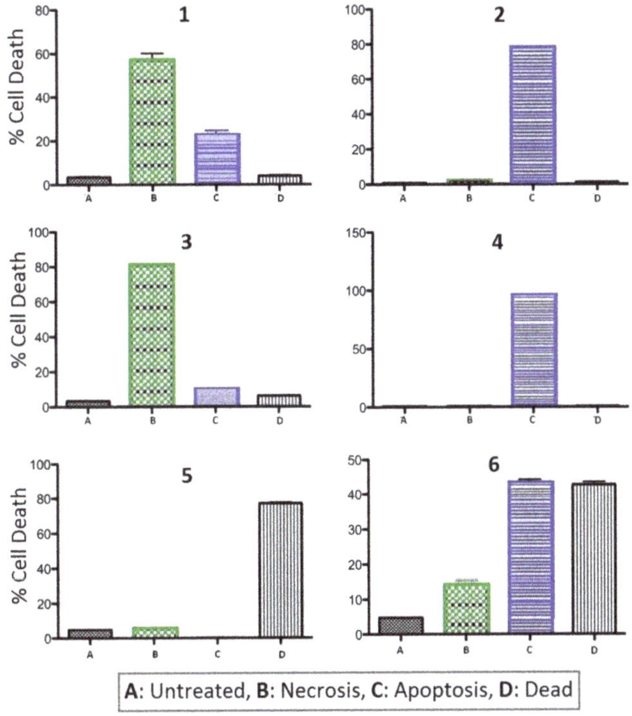

Figure 4. Summary plots of flow cytometry data using Annexin V-FITC and PI to determine mode of cell death for **1–6** (necrotic PI^+/AnV^-; apoptotic PI^-/AnV^+; dead/late apoptosis PI^+/AnV^-).

2.2.3. *In Vitro* Cytotoxicity Screening at the NCI

With the discovery that **1**/**3** and **2**/**4** exhibit contrasting mechanisms of cell death towards Jurkat cells, the set of **1–6** were further screened for *in vitro* antitumor activity at the National Cancer Institute [10]. In one dose (10 μM) testing, dioxothiazine regioisomers **3** and **4** exhibited more potent panel average cell kill than the natural products **1** and **2**, with precursor quinones **5** and **6** being found to be the least active (see Supplementary Materials). Selectivity towards melanoma cell lines, in particular MDA-MB-435 (all compounds) and MALME-3M (**3** and **4**), was observed. More comprehensive

5-dose testing of **1–4** identified **3**, the regioisomer of thiaplidiaquinone A, to be the more active compound, showing good activity towards MDA-MB-435 (LC_{50} 0.66 μM, TGI 0.18 μM, GI_{50} 0.052 μM) and MALME-3M (LC_{50} 3.4 μM, TGI 0.60 μM, GI_{50} 0.10 μM) cell lines (see Supplementary Materials). This compound has been selected for further *in vivo* evaluation. Our findings that non-natural dioxothiazine regioisomers can exhibit more potent cytotoxicity to tumour cells than the corresponding natural product is in agreement with results observed by Aiello *et al.*, as part of their SAR studies of the dioxothiazine-ring containing ascidian natural product aplidinone A [11]. Their study investigated the effect of variation in lipophilic sidechain structure and dioxothiazine ring regiochemistry on a range of biological activities. They identified one structurally simplified analogue of the natural product containing the non-natural dioxothiazine ring regiochemistry that exhibited enhanced cytotoxicity towards a number of tumour cell lines as well as enhanced inhibition of TNFα-induced Nf-κB activation.

2.2.4. Antimalarial and Anti-Farnesyltransferase Activities

Compounds **1–6** were evaluated for activity against *Plasmodium falciparum* (NF54 chloroquine sensitive and FcM29-Cameroon chloroquine-resistant strains) and protozoal and human protein farnesyltransferases. The results are presented in Table 1. We have previously determined that the structurally-related marine meroterpene scabellone B exhibited moderate antimalarial activity (IC_{50} 4.8 μM, *Pf* K1 strain) [3]. Evaluation of **1–6** against *P. falciparum* identified precursor quinones **5** and **6** to be the most active, followed by regioisomers **3** and **4**, while natural products **1** and **2** were deemed inactive. We have previously determined that the structurally-related marine meroterpene scabellone B exhibited moderate antimalarial activity (IC_{50} 4.8 μM, *Pf* K1 strain). [3] Taken together, these results show that compounds containing only the tricyclic pyranoquinone core structure (*i.e.*, rings B-C-D) such as in compounds **5**, **6** and scabellone B are more active antimalarial agents than those compounds that also contain an additional dioxothiazine ring. The results also suggest that amongst the dioxothiazine-containing compounds **1–4**, anti-*Pf* activity is sensitive to the particular regiochemistry of the dioxothiazine ring. With regard to the protein farnesyltransferase (FTase) bioassays, a high degree of correlation was observed between results for FTases of both protozoal and human origin for most of the compounds. In the cases of compounds **2** and **6**, a slightly higher degree of selectivity for human FTase was observed. Of note was the sub-micromolar inhibition of both FTases by the natural product thiaplidiaquinone A (**1**) and regioisomeric analogues **3** and **4**, with the latter exhibiting particularly potent activities (IC_{50} 0.098 and 0.054 μM).

Table 1. *In vitro* antimalarial and anti-farnesyltransferase activity of compounds **1–6**.

Compound	*P. falc.* [a]	FTase (*T. b.*) [b]	FTase (H) [c]
1	>17 [d]	0.74 ± 0.20	0.78 ± 0.17
2	>17 [d]	3.04 ± 0.30	1.22± 0.068
3	4.56 ± 0.76 [d]	0.22 ± 0.034	0.14 ± 0.0017
4	4.39 ± 0.77 [d]	0.098 ± 0.008	0.054 ± 0.005
5	2.2 [e]	3.90 ± 0.60	3.70 ± 0.60
6	2.3 [e]	6.16 ± 1.40	1.64 ± 0.30
Chloroquine [f]	0.45 [d], 0.0063 [e]		
FTI 276 [f]		0.010 ± 0.002	0.015 ± 0.004

IC_{50} values (μM) are reported as the average of three assays with an associated deviation, except for *Pf* data for **5** and **6** which is reported as the average of two independent assays; [a] *Plasmodium falciparum*; [b] *Trypanosoma brucei* farnesyltransferase; [c] Human farnesyltransferase; [d] *Plasmodium falciparum*, FcM29-Cameroon strain (chloroquine-resistant); [e] *Plasmodium falciparum*, NF54 strain (chloroquine sensitive), IEF stage; [f] Chloroquine and FTI 276 were used as positive controls.

3. Experimental Section

3.1. *Chemistry*

The syntheses of compounds **1–6** have been reported previously [5].

3.2. *Biology*

3.2.1. Cell Culture

Jurkat cells were maintained in RPMI 1640 supplemented with 10% FBS, 1% glutamax and 1% Penicillin/streptomycin. Cultures were maintained at 37 °C with 5% CO_2, and split 2–3 times per week.

3.2.2. Intracellular ROS

Cells were resuspended in HBSS at 1×10^6 cells/mL and 100 μL cells added to individual wells of a 96-well round bottom plate. DHR123 was added to the wells for a final concentration of 500 nM per well and cells incubated for 5 min to allow uptake of DHR123. Compounds were made up in DMSO to 10 mM for a stock solution. A ten-fold dilution series was made for each stock solution in HBSS from 1 mM to 10 nM and 10 μL of each added to triplicate wells, for final concentrations of 100 μM to 1 nM, along with corresponding DMSO controls. The assay was incubated at 37 °C for 30 min, and the cells were washed and resuspended in FACS buffer (PBS with 0.1% BSA and 0.2% sodium azide). Intracellular ROS was measured by flow cytometry analysis of DHR123 uptake.

3.2.3. Jurkat Cell Cytotoxicity Assay

Cells were resuspended in cRPMI at 1×10^6 cells/mL and 100 μL cells added to individual wells of a 96-well round bottom plate. Compounds were made up in DMSO to 10 mM for a stock solution. A ten-fold dilution series was made for each stock solution in cRPMI from 1 mM to 10 nM and 10 μL of each added to triplicate wells, for final concentrations of 100 μM to 1 nM, along with corresponding DMSO controls. The cells plus compounds were then incubated for 24 h at 37 °C. The cells were washed in ice-cold Annexin V binding buffer (200 mL PBS with 10 mM HEPES, 140 mM NaCl and 2.5 mM $CaCl_2$). The cell pellets were labelled with 5 μL of Annexin V-FITC (BD Pharmingen) for 15 min at 4 °C. Cells were washed again with ice-cold Annexin V buffer and labelled with 10 μL of 5 μg/mL PI for 7 min at 4 °C. Cells were washed and resuspended in FACS buffer, and Annexin V/PI staining analysed using flow cytometry. Annexin V positive cells were undergoing apoptosis, while PI positive cells were necrotic. Double positive cells were dead, while double negative cells were live cells.

3.2.4. NCI Evaluation

Detailed protocols have been reported elsewhere [12].

3.2.5. Antimalarial and Anti-Farnesyltransferase Evaluation

Detailed protocols have been reported elsewhere [13,14].

4. Conclusions

Our biological evaluation of members of a small library of compounds focused on the marine meroterpenoids thiaplidiaquinone A and B has revealed that the non-natural dioxothiazine regioisomers **3** and **4** tend to exhibit more potent biological activities against a number of cellular targets. An unexpected discovery was that the mechanism of Jurkat cell death was dominantly *via* necrosis for thiaplidiaquinone A but *via* apoptosis for the geranyl sidechain positional isomer thiaplidiaquinone B. The finding that the dioxothiazine regioisomers of the natural products exhibited more potent activities in a range of bioassays highlights the crucial role that total synthesis can play in the discovery of new bioactive scaffolds.

Acknowledgments: We acknowledge funding from the University of Auckland and Marcel Kaiser of Swiss Tropical and Public Health Institute for antimalarial data for compounds **5** and **6**.

Author Contributions: B.C., D.B., M.-L.B.-K. and J.H. conceived and designed the experiments; L.S., J.H., J.D. and A.V. performed the experiments; I.K. synthesized the compounds; J.H., M.-L.B.-K., J.D., A.V. and B.C. analyzed the data; and all authors contributed to writing the paper.

Conflicts of Interest: The authors declare no conflict of interest.

References

1. Zubía, E.; Ortega, M.J.; Salvá, J. Natural products chemistry in marine ascidians of the genus *Aplidium*. *Mini Rev. Org. Chem.* **2005**, *2*, 389–399.
2. Appleton, D.R.; Chuen, C.S.; Berridge, M.V.; Webb, V.L.; Copp, B.R. Rossinones A and B, biologically active meroterpenoids from the Antarctic ascidian, *Aplidium* species. *J. Org. Chem.* **2009**, *74*, 9195–9198.
3. Chan, S.T.S.; Pearce, A.N.; Januario, A.H.; Page, M.J.; Kaiser, M.; McLaughlin, R.J.; Harper, J.L.; Webb, V.L.; Barker, D.; Copp, B.R. Anti-inflammatory and antimalarial meroterpenoids from the New Zealand ascidian *Aplidium scabellum*. *J. Org. Chem.* **2011**, *76*, 9151–9156.
4. Aiello, A.; Fattorusso, E.; Luciano, P.; Macho, A.; Menna, M.; Muñoz, E. Antitumor effects of two novel naturally occurring terpene quinones isolated from the Mediterranean ascidian *Aplidium conicum*. *J. Med. Chem.* **2005**, *48*, 3410–3416.
5. Khalil, I.M.; Barker, D.; Copp, B.R. Biomimetic synthesis of thiaplidiaquinones A and B. *J. Nat. Prod.* **2012**, *75*, 2256–2260.
6. Carbone, A.; Lucas, C.L.; Moody, C.J. Biomimetic synthesis of the apoptosis-inducing thiazinoquinone thiaplidiaquinone A. *J. Org. Chem.* **2012**, *77*, 9179–9189.
7. Emmendorffer, A.; Hecht, M.; Lohmann-Matthes, M.-L.; Roesler, J. A fast and easy method to determine the production of reactive oxygen intermediates by human and murine phagocytes using dihydrorhodamine 123. *J. Immunol. Methods* **1990**, *131*, 269–275.
8. Villena, J.; Henriquez, M.; Torres, V.; Moraga, F.; Diaz-Elizondo, J.; Arredondo, C.; Chiong, M.; Olea-Azar, C.; Stutzin, A.; Lavandero, S.; *et al.* Ceramide-induced formation of ROS and ATP depletion trigger necrosis in lymphoid cells. *Free Radic. Biol. Med.* **2008**, *44*, 1146–1160.
9. Maschke, M.; Alborzinia, H.; Lieb, M.; Wolfl, S.; Metzler-Nolte, N. Structure-activity relationship of trifluoromethyl-containing metallocenes: Electrochemistry, lipophilicity, cytotoxicity, and ROS production. *ChemMedChem* **2014**, *9*, 1188–1194. [PubMed]
10. Shoemaker, R.H. The NCI60 human tumour cell line anticancer drug screen. *Nat. Rev. Cancer* **2006**, *6*, 813–823. [PubMed]
11. Aiello, A.; Fattorusso, E.; Luciano, P.; Menna, M.; Calzado, M.A.; Muñoz, E.; Bonadies, F.; Guiso, M.; Sanasi, M.F.; Cocco, G.; *et al.* Synthesis of structurally simplified analogues of aplidinone A, a pro-apoptotic marine thiazinoquinone. *Bioorg. Med. Chem.* **2010**, *18*, 719–727. [CrossRef]
12. Boyd, M.R.; Paull, K.D. Some practical considerations and applications of the National Cancer Institute *in vitro* anticancer drug discovery screen. *Drug Dev. Res.* **1995**, *34*, 91–109. [CrossRef]
13. Longeon, A.; Copp, B.R.; Roué, M.; Dubois, J.; Valentin, A.; Petek, S.; Debitus, C.; Bourguet-Kondracki, M.-L. New bioactive halenaquinone derivatives from South Pacific marine sponges of the genus *Xestospongia*. *Bioorg. Med. Chem.* **2010**, *18*, 6006–6011. [CrossRef] [PubMed]
14. Ménan, H.; Banzouzi, J.-T.; Hocquette, A.; Pélissier, Y.; Blache, Y.; Koné, M.; Mallié, M.; Assi, L.A.; Valentin, A. Antiplasmodial activity and cytotoxicity of plants used in West African traditional medicine for the treatment of malaria. *J. Ethnopharmacol.* **2006**, *105*, 131–136. [CrossRef] [PubMed]

marine drugs

MDPI

Article

Isolation and Total Synthesis of Stolonines A–C, Unique Taurine Amides from the Australian Marine Tunicate *Cnemidocarpa stolonifera*

Trong D. Tran [1], Ngoc B. Pham [1], Merrick Ekins [2], John N. A. Hooper [1,2] and Ronald J. Quinn [1,*]

[1] Eskitis Institute for Drug Discovery, Griffith University, Brisbane, Queensland 4111, Australia; trong.tran@griffithuni.edu.au (T.D.T.); n.pham@griffith.edu.au (N.B.P.); john.hooper@qm.qld.gov.au (J.N.A.H.)

[2] Queensland Museum, Brisbane, Queensland 4101, Australia; merrick.ekins@qm.qld.gov.au

[*] Author to whom correspondence should be addressed; r.quinn@griffith.edu.au; Tel.: +61-7-3735-6009; Fax: +61-7-3735-6001.

Academic Editor: Sylvia Urban

Received: 19 June 2015; Accepted: 14 July 2015; Published: 22 July 2015

Abstract: *Cnemidocarpa stolonifera* is an underexplored marine tunicate that only occurs on the tropical to subtropical East Coast of Australia, with only two pyridoacridine compounds reported previously. Qualitative analysis of the lead-like enhanced fractions of C. *stolonifera* by LC-MS dual electrospray ionization coupled with PDA and ELSD detectors led to the identification of three new natural products, stolonines A–C (**1–3**), belonging to the taurine amide structure class. Structures of the new compounds were determined by NMR and MS analyses and later verified by total synthesis. This is the first time that the conjugates of taurine with 3-indoleglyoxylic acid, quinoline-2-carboxylic acid and β-carboline-3-carboxylic acid present in stolonines A–C (**1–3**), respectively, have been reported. An immunofluorescence assay on PC3 cells indicated that compounds **1** and **3** increased cell size, induced mitochondrial texture elongation, and *caused apoptosis in PC3 cells.*

Keywords: *Cnemidocarpa stolonifera*; taurine amide; PC3 cell line; immunofluorescence assay

1. Introduction

The exploration of marine secondary metabolites only began in the early 1950s [1] with the landmark identification of the two nucleosides spongothymidine and spongouridine from the Caribbean marine sponge *Cryptotethia crypta* [2,3]. Since then, marine natural product discovery has increased annually and has accelerated over the last two decades [4]. By 2010 more than 15,000 new marine natural products were discovered with 8368 new compounds recorded in a decade between 2001 and 2010 [5]. Approximately 75% of marine natural products were isolated from marine invertebrates [4] from which sponges, tunicates, bryozoans or molluscs have provided the majority of the compounds involved in clinical or preclinical trials [5]. It is expected that the discovery of marine natural products will provide new and improved therapeutics for human illnesses, along with other innovative products for other industrial activities (e.g., nutraceutics and biotechnology) [6].

To maximize the chance to discover new marine natural products, a library of fractions from rare or restricted marine invertebrates was generated from the Nature Bank database [7]. Qualitative analysis of lead-like enhanced fractions of samples in the selected library by LC-MS dual electrospray ionization coupled with PDA and ELSD detectors [8–10] indicated that the marine tunicate *Cnemidocarpa stolonifera* contained two different compound classes in two different fractions. The first class showed strong MS signals in a positive mode and strong UV absorptions at 380 nm while the second one displayed strong MS signals in a negative mode and strong UV absorptions at 280 nm. Mass-guided isolation of the marine tunicate *C. stolonifera* extract led to the isolation of two known pyridoacridine alkaloids, 11-hydroxyascididemin (**4**) and cnemidine A (**5**) [11], accounting for the first compound class. For the second class of compounds, three new taurine amide derivatives, stolonines A–C (**1–3**), were isolated.

Taurine is found at high concentration in mammalian plasma and tissues [12]. This compound has been known to exhibit a large spectrum of physiological functions in the liver, kidney, heart, pancreas, retina, and brain [13,14]. Its depletion is associated with several disease conditions such as diabetes, Parkinson's, Alzheimer's, cardiovascular diseases, and neuronal damages in the retina [13]. So far, 81 taurine derivatives from natural sources have been reported of which 47 compounds are amides produced between taurine with fatty acids, steroid acids or other aromatic acid residues [15]. The occurrence of the conjugates of taurine with 3-indoleglyoxylic acid, quinoline-2-carboxylic acid and β-carboline-3-carboxylic acid present in stolonines A–C (**1–3**), respectively, has not been previously reported. This paper describes the isolation, structure elucidation and total synthesis of stolonines A–C (**1–3**) from the marine tunicate *C. stolonifera*. Cytotoxicity of **1–3** against human prostate cancer PC3 cell line was evaluated and the result indicated that they were not active up to 20 μM. However, an immunofluorescence assay on PC3 cells revealed that compounds **1** and **3** increased cell size, induced mitochondrial texture elongation and caused apoptosis in PC3 cells.

2. Results and Discussion

The freeze-dried *C. stolonifera* tunicate was sequentially extracted with *n*-hexane, dichloromethane (DCM), and methanol (MeOH). The DCM/MeOH extracts were then combined and chromatographed using C_{18} bonded silica HPLC MeOH/H_2O/0.1% trifluoroacetic acid (TFA) to yield three new alkaloids, stolonines A–C (**1–3**) together with two known alkaloids, 11-hydroxyascididemin (**4**) and cnemidine A (**5**) (Figure 1).

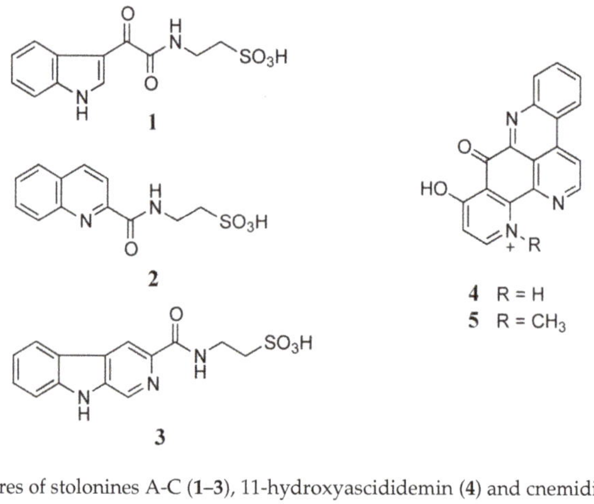

Figure 1. Structures of stolonines A-C (**1–3**), 11-hydroxyascididemin (**4**) and cnemidine A (**5**) isolated from the tunicate *C. stolonifera*.

Stolonine A (**1**) was obtained as a white amorphous solid. The (−)-HRESIMS spectrum displayed a molecular ion $[M-H]^-$ at m/z 295.0390, which was consistent with the molecular formula $C_{12}H_{12}N_2O_5S$. The IR spectrum indicated the presence of an S=O stretching band at 1205 cm^{-1} [16]. A ^{1}H NMR spectrum of **1** showed two exchangeable protons (δ_H 12.20 and 8.78 ppm), five aromatic protons (δ_H 8.82, 8.22, 7.52, 7.26 and 7.24 ppm) and two methylenes (δ_H 3.50 and 2.66 ppm). Further analysis of the ^{13}C NMR and gHSQCAD spectra indicated that the molecule contained two carbonyls (δ_C 181.6 and 162.7 ppm), eight aromatic carbons (δ_C 138.5, 136.2, 126.2, 123.3, 122.4, 121.3, 112.5 and 112.1 ppm) and two methylenes (δ_C 49.8 and 35.5 ppm) (Table 1). *J* coupling constants of aromatic protons H-4 (δ_H 8.22, dd, 1.8, 7.2 Hz), H-5 (δ_H 7.24, dt, 1.8, 7.2 Hz), H-6 (δ_H 7.26, dt, 1.8, 7.2 Hz) and H-7 (δ_H 7.52, dd, 1.8, 7.2 Hz) and their COSY correlations were characteristic of a 1,2-disubstituted benzene ring (**a**, Figure 2). A gCOSY spectrum displayed correlations from the exchangeable proton H-1 (δ_H 12.20, br.s) to H-2 (δ_H 8.82, d, 3.0 Hz) and also from H-11 (δ_H 3.50, dd, 6.0, 6.6 Hz) to the triplet exchangeable proton H-10 (δ_H 8.78, t, 5.4 Hz) and H-12 (δ_H 2.66, t, 6.6 Hz) facilitating the establishment of two other spin systems, –NH–CH= (**b**, Figure 2) and –NH–CH2–CH2– (**c**, Figure 2) respectively. The aromatic carbon C-3 (δ_C 112.1 ppm) was attached to C-2 (δ_C 138.5 ppm) in the moiety **b** determined by a HMBC correlation from H-2 to C-3. A HMBC correlation from H-2 to C-7a (δ_C 136.2 ppm) supported the linkage from **a** to **b** at C-7a (Figure 2). Both protons H-10 and H-11 in the moiety **c** showed HMBC correlations with a carbonyl carbon at δ_C 162.7 ppm suggesting the connection of this carbonyl to N-10 to form an amide bond (**c**, Figure 2). Two methylene signals at δ_H 3.50 and 2.66 ppm corresponding to carbons C-11 (δ_C 35.5 ppm) and C-12 (δ_C 49.8 ppm) as well as the relatively downfield resonance of the methylene C-12 were diagnostic of methylenes in a taurine moiety (**c**, Figure 2) [17–19].

Table 1. NMR data for **1** in DMSO-d_6 [a].

Position	δ_C	δ_H (J in Hz)	gCOSY	gHMBCAD
1		12.20, br.s	2	
2	138.5	8.82, d (3.0)	1	3, 3a, 7a
3	112.1			
3a	126.2			
4	121.3	8.22, dd (1.8, 7.2)	5	6, 7a
5	122.4	7.24, dt (1.8, 7.2)	4, 6	3a, 7
6	123.3	7.26, dt (1.8, 7.2)	5, 7	4, 7a
7	112.5	7.52, dd (1.8, 7.2)	6	3a, 5
7a	136.2			
8	181.6			
9	162.7			
10		8.78, t (5.4)	11	9
11	35.5	3.50, dd (6.0, 6.6)	10, 12	9, 12
12	49.8	2.66, t (6.6)	11	11

[a] ^{1}H NMR at 600 MHz referenced to residual DMSO solvent (δ_H 2.50 ppm) and ^{13}C NMR at 150 MHz referenced to residual DMSO solvent (δ_C 39.52 ppm).

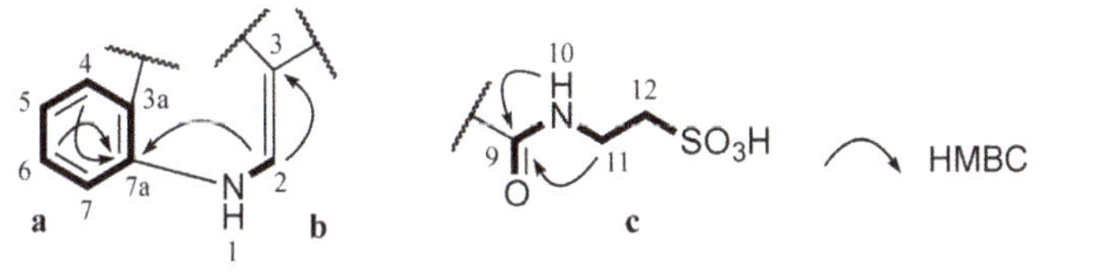

Figure 2. Partial structures (**a**, **b** and **c**) of **1** and their key HMBC correlations.

No HMBC correlation from any proton to the carbonyl C-8 (δ_C 181.6 ppm) was observed when HMBC experiments were performed and optimized with different J_{HC} couplings. Therefore, two different isomers **1-I** and **1-II** were conceivable from these data (Figure 3). Detailed HMBC analysis showed that H-2 had a HMBC correlation with C-3a (δ_C 126.2 ppm). This suggested that **1** was favorable to **1-I** since the H-2 to C-3a correlation in **1-I** was a three-bond coupling while the H-2 to C-3a correlation in **1-II** was a four-bond coupling (Figure 3).

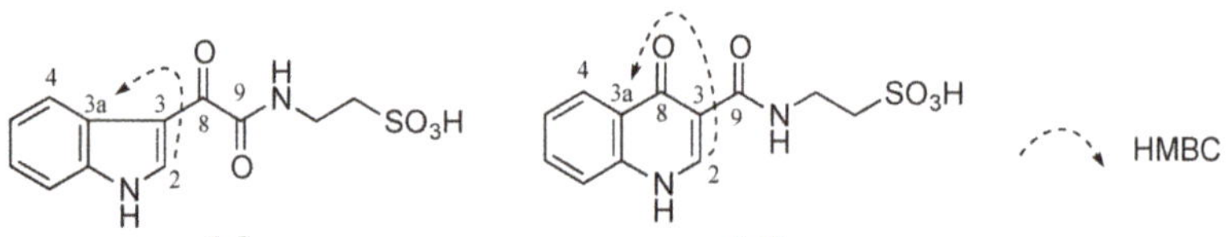

1-I **1-II**

Figure 3. Two possible structures **1-I** and **1-II** of **1** (**1-I** and **1-II** are possible structural isomers of **1**).

Density functional theory (DFT) NMR calculations together with the DP4 probability analysis, which have recently emerged as powerful tools for the determination of structures that lack sufficient NMR characterization or contain unusual constituents or connectivities [20–25], were employed to verify the assigned structure for **1**. Theoretical ^{1}H and ^{13}C chemical shifts were calculated at the mPW1PW91/6-31G(d)//B3lyp/6-31G(d) levels. Calculated NMR data of **1-I** and **1-II** were then compared with the experimental NMR data based on the corrected mean absolute error (CMAE) and the DP4 probability (Computational Details, Experimental Section) to determine which of the isomers fit with the experimental data. The results (Table 2) indicated that both ^{13}C and ^{1}H chemical shifts of the isomer **1-I** showed lower CMAE compared to those of the isomer **1-II**. Significant differences were observed in DP4 probabilities. In particular, **1-I** had 100% probability for ^{13}C chemical shifts and 85.3% probability for ^{1}H chemical shifts while **1-II** only occupied 0% for ^{13}C chemical shifts and 14.7% for ^{1}H chemical shifts (Table 2). These probabilities indicated that the assignment of the isomer **1-I** for **1** was at a high level of confidence [20]. Therefore, the structure of **1** was suggested as the isomer **1-I**.

Table 2. Comparison of experimental and calculated ^{13}C and ^{1}H chemical shifts for **1** in DMSO-d_6.

Position	**δ_C (Exp.)**	**1-I**		**1-II**		**δ_H (Exp.)**	**1-I**		**1-II**	
		δ_C (Calc.)	**δ_C (Scaled)**	**δ_C (Calc.)**	**δ_C (Scaled)**		**δ_H (Calc.)**	**δ_H (Scaled)**	**δ_H (Calc.)**	**δ_H (Scaled)**
2	138.5	136.9	140.3	141.3	142.8	8.82	8.74	8.61	8.84	8.67
3	112.1	111.5	112.9	111.2	110.2					
3a	126.2	124.1	126.5	123.0	122.9					
4	121.3	118.9	120.9	124.3	124.4	8.22	8.62	8.48	8.40	8.19
5	122.4	120.1	122.1	121.1	120.9	7.24	7.63	7.40	7.63	7.35
6	123.3	120.9	123.0	129.4	129.9	7.26	7.59	7.36	8.00	7.76
7	112.5	108.7	109.9	114.8	114.1	7.52	7.55	7.31	7.53	7.24
7a	136.2	131.9	134.9	134.4	135.3					
8	181.6	176.7	183.2	172.5	176.5					
9	162.7	156.8	161.7	159.4	162.4					
11	35.5	37.1	32.6	36.9	29.8	3.50	3.69	3.11	3.71	3.08
12	49.8	57.2	54.4	58.4	53.1	2.66	3.55	2.95	3.57	2.93
CMAE			1.5		3.1			0.23		0.25
DP4		100.0%		0.0%			85.3%		14.7%	

Compound **1-I** was synthesized by coupling 3-indoleglyoxylic acid (**6**) with taurine (Scheme 1) in the presence of *N*-(3-dimethylaminopropyl)-*N′*-ethylcarbodiimide (EDCI), *N*-hydroxybenzotriazole (HOBt) and dimethylformamide (DMF) at room temperature (rt) for 21 h (64% yield) [26]. Both ^{1}H and ^{13}C NMR data of the synthetic **1-I** completely matched those of the natural product **1** (Table 3) confirming that **1-I** was the structure of **1**. Therefore, compound **1** was defined as a new alkaloid with a trivial name stolonine A.

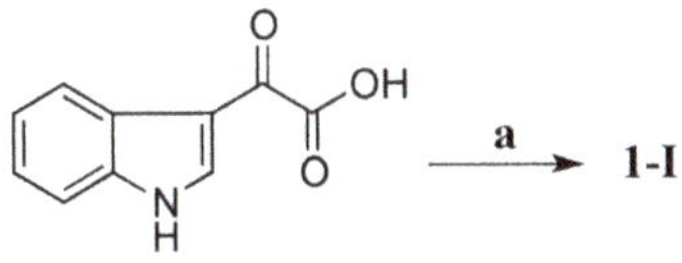

6

Scheme 1. Synthesis of **1**. (**a**) Taurine, EDCI, HOBt, DMF, rt, 21 h, 64%.

Table 3. ^{1}H and ^{13}C NMR chemical shifts of natural and synthetic products of **1–3** [a].

Position	1				2				3			
	Natural Product [a]		Synthetic Product [b]		Natural Product [a]		Synthetic Product [b]		Natural Product [a]		Synthetic Product [b]	
	δ_C	δ_H (*J* in Hz)	δ_C	δ_H (*J* in Hz)	δ_C	δ_H (*J* in Hz)	δ_C [a]	δ_H (*J* in Hz)	δ_C	δ_H (*J* in Hz)	δ_C	δ_H (*J* in Hz)
1		12.20, br.s		12.19, br.s					131.3	8.95, s	131.3	8.95, s
2	138.5	8.82, d (3.0)	138.5	8.82, d (3.0)	150.1		150.1					
3	112.1		112.1		118.6	8.15, d (8.4)	118.6	8.15, d (8.5)	138.0		138.0	
3a	126.2		126.2									
4	121.3	8.22, dd (1.8, 7.2)	121.3	8.22, d (7.5)	137.8	8.55, d (8.4)	137.8	8.55, d (8.5)	114.0	8.93, s	114.1	8.93, s
4a					129.2		129.2		128.9		129.0	
4b									120.7		120.7	
5	122.4	7.24, dt (1.8, 7.2)	122.4	7.24, t (7.5)	128.7	8.08, d (7.8)	128.7	8.08, d (8.0)	122.3	8.39, d (7.8)	122.3	8.39, d (8.0)
6	123.3	7.26, dt (1.8, 7.2)	123.3	7.26, t (7.5)	128.0	7.71, t (7.2, 7.8)	128.0	7.71, t (8.0)	120.3	7.35, t (7.2, 7.8)	120.3	7.35, t (7.5, 8.0)
7	112.5	7.52, dd (1.8, 7.2)	112.5	7.52, d (7.5)	130.4	7.87, t (7.2, 7.8)	130.4	7.87, t (8.0)	129.2	7.64, t (7.2, 7.8)	129.2	7.64, t (7.5, 8.0)
7a	136.2		136.2									
8	181.6		181.6		128.1	8.06, d (7.8)	128.1	8.06, d (8.0)	112.5	7.70, d (7.8)	112.5	7.70, d (8.0)
8a					146.0		146.0		141.6		141.6	
9	162.7		162.7		163.5		163.5			12.11, s		12.10, s
9a									136.7		136.6	
10		8.78, t (5.4)		8.78, t (5.4)		9.29, t (5.4)		9.29, t (5.0)	163.3		163.3	
11	35.5	3.50, dd (6.0, 6.6)	35.5	3.50, dd (6.0, 6.5)	35.9	3.65, dd (6.0, 6.6)	35.9	3.65, dd (5.5, 6.5)		9.15, t (5.4)		9.15, t (5.5)
12	49.8	2.66, t (6.6)	49.8	2.66, t (6.5)	50.1	2.72, t (6.6)	50.1	2.72, t (6.5)	35.9	3.66, dd (5.4, 6.6)	35.9	3.66, dd (5.5, 6.0)
13									50.3	2.72, t (6.6)	50.3	2.72, t (6.0)

[a] ^{1}H NMR at 600 MHz at 30 °C referenced to residual DMSO solvent (δ_H 2.50 ppm) and ^{13}C NMR at 150 MHz at 30 °C referenced to residual DMSO solvent (δ_C 39.52 ppm); [b] ^{1}H NMR at 500 MHz at 30 °C referenced to residual DMSO solvent (δ_H 2.50 ppm) and ^{13}C NMR at 125 MHz at 30 °C referenced to residual DMSO solvent (δ_C 39.52 ppm).

Stolonine B (**2**) was purified as a white amorphous solid. A molecular ion $[M - H]^-$ at *m/z* 279.0441 in the (−)-HRESIMS spectrum indicated that **2** had a molecular formula $C_{12}H_{12}N_2O_4S$. A ^{1}H NMR spectrum of **2** displayed one exchangeable proton (δ_H 9.29 ppm), six aromatic protons (δ_H 8.55, 8.15, 8.08, 8.06, 7.87 and 7.71 ppm) and two methylenes (δ_H 3.65 and 2.72 ppm). ^{13}C NMR combined with gHSQCAD spectra indicated that **2** contained nine aromatic carbons including six tertiary carbons (δ_C 137.8, 130.4, 128.7, 128.1, 128.0 and 118.6 ppm) and three quaternary carbons (δ_C 150.1, 146.0 and 129.2 ppm), one carbonyl (δ_C 163.5 ppm) and two methylenes (δ_C 50.1 and 35.9 ppm) (Table 4). Compared to **1**, compound **2** displayed similar COSY and HMBC correlations from the two methylene protons resulting in the assignment of a taurine moiety. A 1,2-disubstituted benzene ring was deduced on the basis of *J* coupling constants and COSY correlations of H-5 (δ_H 8.08, d, 7.8 Hz), H-6 (δ_H 7.71, t, 7.2, 7.8 Hz), H-7 (δ_H 7.87, t, 7.2, 7.8 Hz) and H-8 (δ_H 8.06, d, 7.8 Hz). Two doublet aromatic protons H-3 (δ_H 8.15 ppm) and H-4 (δ_H 8.55 ppm) coupling together with a *J* coupling value of 8.4 Hz showed HMBC correlations from H-3 to C-4a (δ_C 129.2 ppm) and from H-4 to C-5 (δ_C 128.7 ppm) and C-8a (δ_C 146.0 ppm) facilitating a connection from **c** to **b** at C-4. Two quaternary carbons C-2 (δ_C 150.1 ppm) and C-8a (δ_C 146.0 ppm) were linked through a nitrogen atom N-1 based on their downfield resonances, which are characteristic for the imine carbons [27]. According to a HMBC correlation from H-4 to the imine C-2, C-2 was attached to C-3 leading to the establishment of a quinoline ring system.

Table 4. NMR data for **2** in DMSO-d_6 [a].

Position	δ_C	δ_H (J in Hz)	gCOSY	gHMBCAD
2	150.1			
3	118.6	8.15, d (8.4)	4	4a
4	137.8	8.55, d (8.4)	3	2, 5, 8a
4a	129.2			
5	128.7	8.08, d (7.8)	6	4, 7, 8a
6	128.0	7.71, t (7.2, 7.8)	5, 7	4a, 8
7	130.4	7.87, t (7.2, 7.8)	6, 8	5, 8a
8	128.1	8.06, d (7.8)	7	4a, 6
8a	146.0			
9	163.5			
10		9.29, t (5.4)	11	
11	35.9	3.65, dd (5.4, 6.6)	10, 12	9, 12
12	50.1	2.72, t (6.6)	11	11

[a] ^{1}H NMR at 600 MHz referenced to residual DMSO solvent (δ_H 2.50 ppm) and ^{13}C NMR at 150 MHz referenced to residual DMSO solvent (δ_C 39.52 ppm).

Due to lack of HMBC correlations from H-3 (δ_H 8.15 ppm) to C-9 (δ_C 163.5 ppm) or from H-10 (δ_H 9.29 ppm) to C-2 to obtain unequivocal evidence of the final structure, total synthesis of **2** was undertaken to verify the structure assignment (Scheme 2). *o*-Nitrobenzaldehyde (**7**) was reduced with 4.5 equivalents (eq.) of iron powder in the presence of 0.05 mol of HCl (aqueous, aq.) in ethanol (EtOH) under reflux in 40 min. Methyl pyruvate and potassium hydroxide powder were then added and the condensation reaction was under reflux in additional 1.5 h to obtain quinoline-2-carboxylic acid (**8**) (55% yield) [28]. This compound was coupled with taurine using EDCI/HOBt in DMF at rt for 48 h to produce **2** with a yield of 75%. The NMR data of the synthetic compound **2** (Table 3) was identical to that of the natural product **2** confirming the structure assignment of **2** as a new taurine amide. Thus, the structure of **2**, stolonine B, was established.

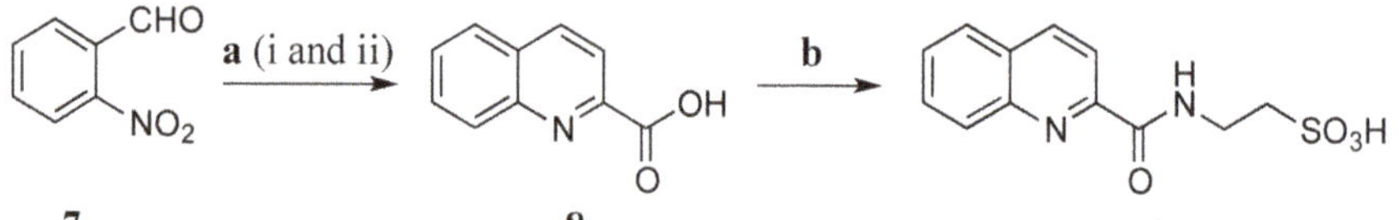

Scheme 2. Synthesis of **2**. (**a**) (i) Fe, HCl, EtOH, reflux, 40 min; (ii) methyl pyruvate, KOH, reflux, 1.5 h, 55% (**b**) Taurine, EDCI, HOBt, DMF, rt, 48 h, 75%.

Stolonine C (**3**) was isolated as a white amorphous solid. Its (−)-HRESIMS spectrum showed a signal for $[M - H]^-$ at m/z 318.0550 indicating a molecular formula $C_{14}H_{13}N_3O_4S$ to be assigned to **3**. A ^{13}C NMR spectrum combined with 2D NMR data indicated that compound **3** had 11 aromatic carbons including six tertiary carbons (δ_C 132.2, 128.2, 122.3, 120.0, 113.9 and 112.3 ppm), five quaternary carbons (δ_C 141.1, 139.6, 137.1, 128.7 and 121.0 ppm), one carbonyl (δ_C 164.3 ppm) and two methylenes (δ_C 50.4 and 35.7 ppm) (Table 5). COSY and HMBC correlations confirmed **3** had a taurine moiety (**a**, Figure 4) and a 1,2-disubstituted benzene ring (**b**, Figure 4), which were similar to those in **1** and **2**. HMBC correlations from a singlet proton H-1 (δ_H 8.89 ppm) to C-3 (δ_C 139.6 ppm), C-4a (δ_C 128.7 ppm) and C-9a (δ_C 137.1 ppm) and from a singlet proton H-4 (δ_H 8.84 ppm) to C-9a indicated the presence of a 2,4,5-trisubstituted pyridine ring (**c**, Figure 4). HMBC correlations from an exchangeable proton H-9 (δ_H 11.96 ppm) to C-4a, C-9a, C-4b (δ_C 121.0 ppm) and C-8a (δ_C 141.1 ppm) supported the connection of **b** to **c** forming a β-carboline ring system. A HMBC key correlation from H-4 to C-10 (δ_C 164.3 ppm) allowed the connection of **c** to **a** at C-3 (δ_C 139.6 ppm). Therefore, the structure of stolonine C (**3**) was determined as shown in Figure 4.

Table 5. NMR data for **3** in DMSO-d_6.

Position	δ_C [a]	δ_H (*J* in Hz) [a]	δ_C [b,c]	δ_H (*J* in Hz) [b]	gCOSY [b]	gHMBCAD [b]
1	132.2	8.89, s	131.3	8.95, s		3, 4a, 9a
3	139.6		138.0			
4	113.9	8.84, s	114.0	8.93, s		4b, 9a, 10
4a	128.7		128.9			
4b	121.0		120.7			
5	122.3	8.39, d (8.1)	122.3	8.39, d (7.8)	6	4a, 7, 8a
6	120.0	7.30, t (7.2, 8.1)	120.3	7.35, t (7.2, 7.8)	5, 7	4b, 8
7	128.2	7.59, t (7.2, 8.1)	129.2	7.64, t (7.2, 7.8)	6, 8	5, 8a
8	112.3	7.65, d (8.1)	112.5	7.70, d (7.8)	7	4b, 6
8a	141.1		141.6			
9		11.96, s		12.11, s		4a, 4b, 8a, 9a
9a	137.1		136.7			
10	164.3		163.3			
11		9.09, t (5.4)		9.15, t (5.4)	12	
12	35.7	3.64, dd (5.4, 6.3)	35.9	3.66, dd (5.4, 6.6)	11, 13	10, 13
13	50.4	2.70, t (6.3)	50.3	2.72, t (6.6)	12	12

[a] ^1H NMR at 900 MHz at 25 °C referenced to residual DMSO solvent (δ_H 2.50 ppm) and ^{13}C NMR at 225 MHz at 25 °C referenced to residual DMSO solvent (δ_C 39.52 ppm); [b] ^1H NMR at 600 MHz at 30 °C referenced to residual DMSO solvent (δ_H 2.50 ppm) and ^{13}C NMR at 150 MHz at 30 °C referenced to residual DMSO solvent (δ_C 39.52 ppm); [c] ^{13}C chemical shifts obtained from correlations observed in gHSQCAD and gHMBCAD spectra.

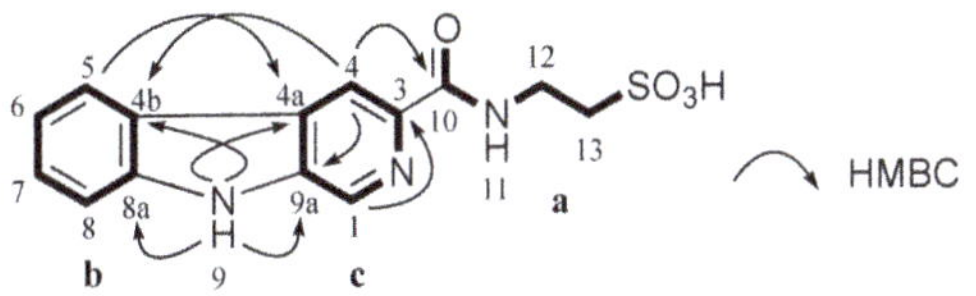

Figure 4. Partial structures (**a**, **b** and **c**) of **3** and their key HMBC correlations.

Total synthesis of **3** was performed using L-tryptophan methyl ester (**9**) as a starting material (Scheme 3). The L-tryptophan methyl ester was treated with formaldehyde (37% aqueous) in a mixture of MeOH and HCl 0.1 N (ratio 10:1) at rt for 16 h to give methyl (3*S*)-1,2,3,4-tetrahydro-β-carboline-3-carboxylate [29]. The crude methyl (3*S*)-1,2,3,4-tetrahydro-β-carboline-3-carboxylate was further oxidized by activated manganese (IV) oxide (MnO_2) in benzene (C_6H_6) under reflux for 5 h yielding a crude methyl β-carboline-3-carboxylate [30]. This ester was then hydrolysed in a mixture of aq. NaOH 20% and MeOH (ratio 1:4) to provide β-carboline-3-carboxylic acid (**10**) (10% yield in three steps) [30]. Amide coupling of **10** and taurine was performed using EDCI/HOBt in DMF at rt in 16 h to produce **3** with a yield of 40%. The synthetic product **3** had superimposable ^1H and ^{13}C NMR data with stolonine C (**3**) confirming its structure assignment (Table 3).

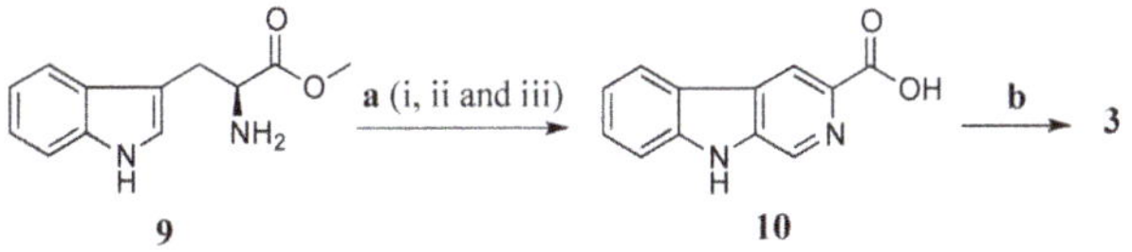

Scheme 3. Synthesis of **3**. (**a**) (i) HCHO, MeOH, HCl 0.1 N, rt, 16 h; (ii) MnO_2, C_6H_6, reflux, 5 h; (iii) NaOH 20%, MeOH, reflux, 45 min (10% in three steps); (**b**) Taurine, EDCI, HOBt, DMF, rt, 16 h, 40%.

Biosynthesis of stolonines A–C (**1–3**) is shown in Scheme 4. Tryptophan (**11**) has been known as a precursor of 3-indoleglyoxylic acid (**6**), quinoline-2-carboxylic acid (**8**) and β-carboline-3-carboxylic acid (**10**) [31]. The acids **6**, **8** and **10** undergo amide bond formation with taurine either by non-ribosomal peptide synthase [32,33] or by acyl-CoA:amino acid *N*-acyltransferase 1 [34,35] to produce stolonines A–C (**1–3**).

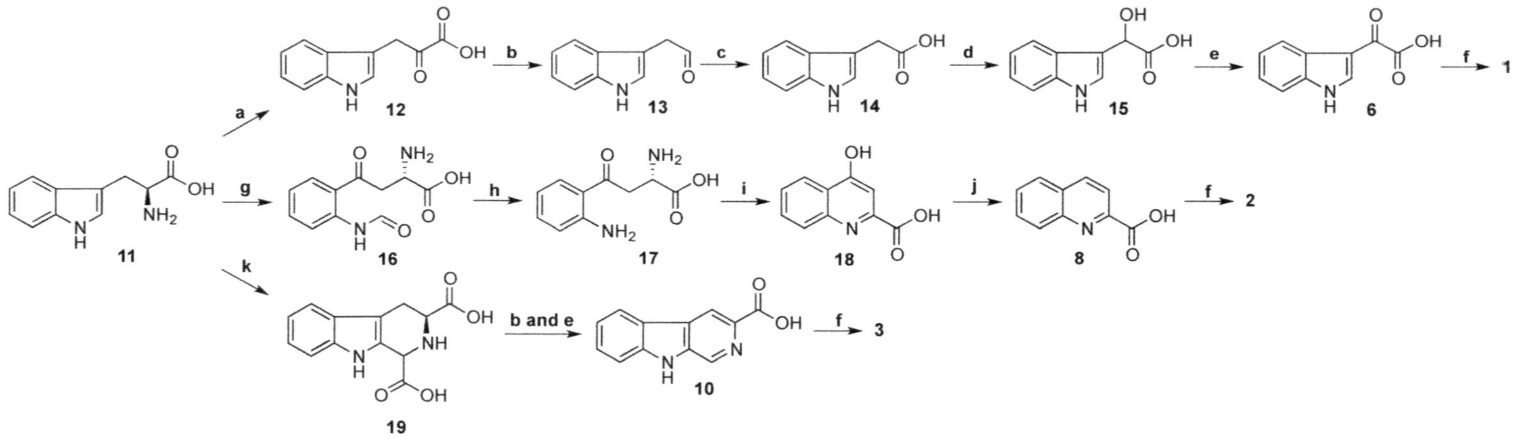

Scheme 4. Biosynthesis of stolonines A–C (**1**–**3**). **a**: transaminase; **b**: decarboxylase; **c**: aldehyde dehydrogenase; **d**: hydroxylase; **e**: dehydrogenase; **f**: taurine + non-ribosomal peptide synthase or acyl-CoA:amino acid *N*-acyltransferase 1; **g**: tryptophan 2,3-dioxygenase or indoleamine 2,3-dioxygenase; **h**: kynurenine formamidase or arylformamidase; **i**: kynurenine aminotransferases; **j**: reductase; **k**: glyoxylic acid.

The two known compounds, 11-hydroxyascididemin (**4**) and cnemidine A (**5**), were identified by NMR comparisons with those in the literature [11].

Cytotoxic evaluation of compounds **1–3** against PC3 cells using the Alamar blue assay indicated that these compounds inhibited the growth of PC3 cells at only 19%, 14%, and 26%, respectively, at their maximum tested concentration of 20 μM. In order to explore whether these compounds have any effect on cellular organelles in PC3 cells, an immunofluorescence assay with three markers for cell membrane, nuclei, and mitochondria was performed. A high-content imaging system was used to image and analyze the data. Compared to vehicle, compounds **1** and **3** had effects on cell morphology, nuclei and mitochondria while compound **2** showed no or very weak effects (Figure 5A). In general, the influence of **1** and **3** on PC3 cells was similar and clearly observed in cell morphology, nuclear, and mitochondrial intensities as well as mitochondrial texture in a dose-dependent manner. In particular, cells treated with **1** and **3** increased cell size and induced cells to become longer shown by the increase in cell, mitochondrial and nuclear area, and the decrease in cell roundness. Compounds **1** and **3** also caused mitochondrial texture to become larger and elongated compared to **2** and DMSO. The increase in nuclear and mitochondrial intensities, which displayed brighter blue-whitish and brighter red-whitish fluorescent appearance respectively in the images (Figure 5B), indicated that the nuclei and mitochondria had more packed masses [36]. The brighter blue-whitish also demonstrated the condensation of chromatins [37], which has been considered as a hallmark feature of apoptotic pathway of programmed cell death [38,39]. The phenotype of nuclei suggested that compounds **1** and **3** affected the PC3 cell death via apoptosis. Moreover, at the non-toxic doses, compounds **1** and **3** also increased the cell size and induced mitochondrial texture elongation. How these compounds influence the PC3 cell morphology and mitochondria is something that warrants further investigation.

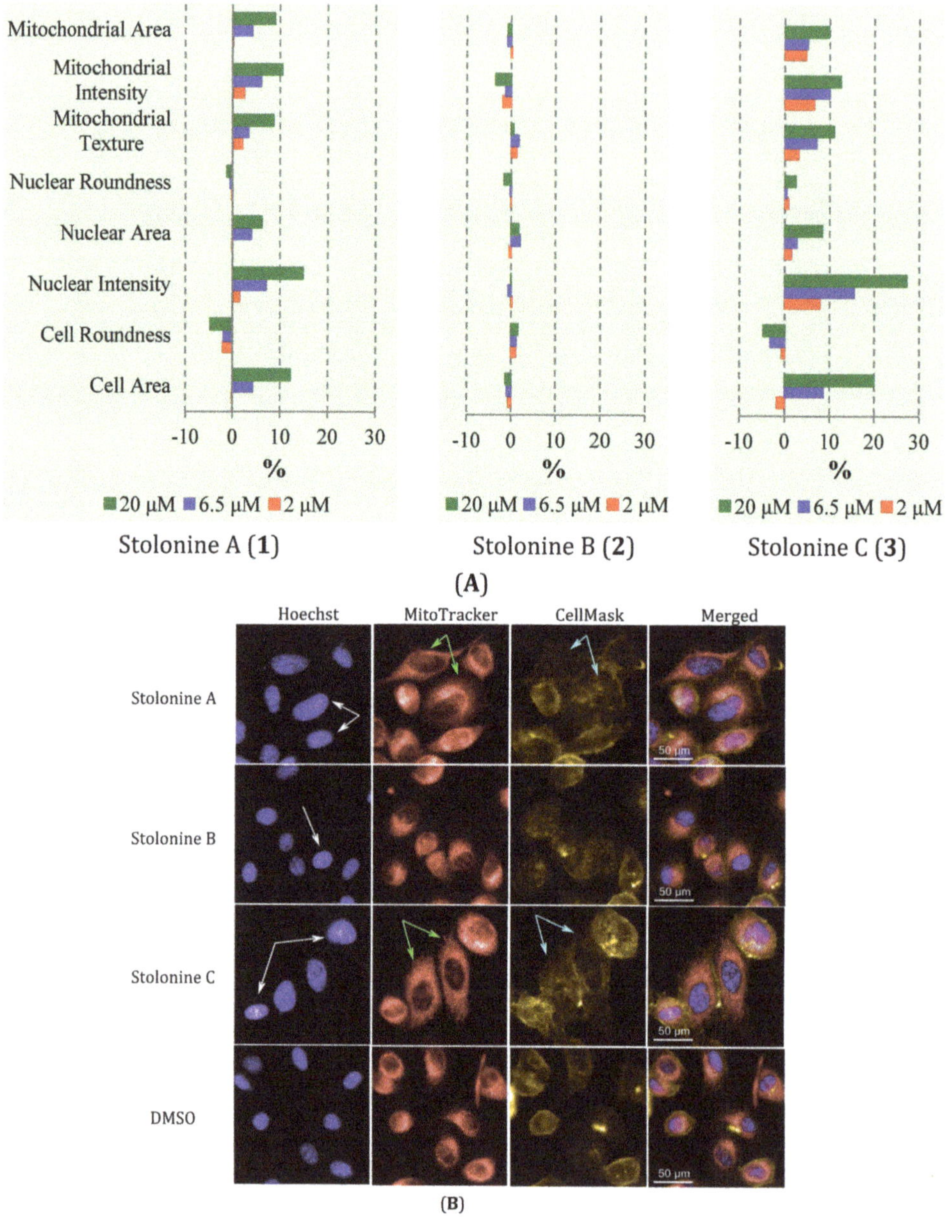

Figure 5. (**A**) Phenotypic profiles for cell proliferation study of **1–3** (results were normalized by a vehicle DMSO); (**B**) Representative images of the PC3 cells treated with 20 μM of **1–3** and DMSO in three channels: Hoechst 33,342 (Blue), MitoTracker (Red) and CellMask (Yellow) (scale bar: 50 μm); chromatin condensation (white arrow), mitochondrial texture elongation (green arrow) and larger cell size (cyan arrow) compared with vehicle DMSO.

3. Experimental Section

3.1. General Experimental Procedures

UV spectra were recorded on a CAMSPEC M501 UV/V is spectrophotometer. NMR spectra were recorded at 30 °C on Varian Inova 500 and 600 MHz and on Bruker 900 MHz spectrometers. The ^{1}H and ^{13}C chemical shifts were referenced to the DMSO-d_6 solvent peaks at δ_H 2.50 and δ_C 39.52 ppm. Standard parameters were used for the 2D NMR spectra obtained, which included gCOSY, gHSQCAD ($^{1}J_{CH}$ = 140 Hz), gHMBCAD ($^{n}J_{CH}$ = 8 Hz), and ROESY. Low-resolution mass spectra were acquired using a Mariner TOF mass spectrometer (Applied Biosystems Pty Ltd, Melbourne, Australia.). High-resolution mass measurement was acquired on a Bruker Solarix 12 Tesla Fourier transform mass spectrometer, fitted with an Apollo API source. For the HPLC isolation, a Water 600 pump equipped with a Water 966 PDA detector and Gilson 715 liquid handler were used. A Betasil C18 column (5 μm, 21.2 × 150 mm) and Hypersil BDS C_{18} column (5 μm, 10 × 250 mm) were used for semi-preparative HPLC. A Phenomenex Luna C_{18} column (3 μm, 4.6 × 50 mm) was used for LC-MS controlled by MassLynx 4.1 software (Waters, Milford, MA, USA). All solvents used for extraction and chromatography were HPLC grade from RCI Labscan or Burdick & Jackson (Lomb Scientific, Sydney, Australia), and the H_2O used was ultrapure water (Arium® proVF, Sartorius Stedim Biotech, Melbourne, Australia).

3.2. Animal Material

A specimen of the tunicate *C. stolonifera* (phylum Tunicata, class Ascidiacea, order Stolidobranchia, family Styelidae) was collected at the depth of 15 m, at Peel Island, Myora Light, North Stradbroke Island, Queensland, Australia in 2005. A voucher specimen (G322208) has been stored at the Queensland Museum, South Brisbane, Queensland, Australia. Material was collected under Moreton Bay Marine Park Permit Number QS2005/CVL588 and Queensland Fisheries Service General Fisheries Permit Number PRM02988B issued to the Queensland Museum.

3.3. Extraction and Isolation

The freeze-dried and ground tunicate *C. stolonifera* (19 g) was extracted exhaustively with hexane (250 mL), DCM (250 mL) and MeOH (2 × 250 mL), respectively. The DCM and MeOH extracts were combined and the solvents were evaporated to yield a yellow residue (2.2 g). This extract was pre-adsorbed onto C_{18} (1 g) and packed dry into a small cartridge, which was connected to a C_{18} preparative HPLC column (5 μm, 21.2 × 150 mm). A linear gradient from 100% H_2O (0.1% TFA) to 100% MeOH (0.1% TFA) was performed over 60 min at a flow rate of 9 mL/min and 60 fractions (1.0 min each) were collected. Pure cnemidine A (**5**, 3.5 mg, 0.018% dry wt) and 11-hydroxyascididemin (**4**, 4.1 mg, 0.021% dry wt) were obtained in fractions 28, 29 and 32 respectively. Fraction 19 was further chromatographed on a Hypersil C_{18} HPLC column (5 μm, 10 × 250 mm) from 10% MeOH (0.1% TFA)/90% H_2O (0.1% TFA) to 25% MeOH (0.1% TFA)/75% H_2O (0.1% TFA) at a flow rate of 4 mL/min in 30 min to yield stolonine C (**3**, 0.1 mg, 0.0021% dry wt) in fraction 14 and stolonine A (**1**, 0.9 mg, 0.0047% dry wt) in fractions 17–18. Fractions 20 and 21 in the first chromatography were combined and purified using the Hypersil C_{18} HPLC column (5 μm, 10 × 250 mm) from 10% MeOH (0.1% TFA)/90% H_2O (0.1% TFA) to 40% MeOH (0.1% TFA)/60% H_2O (0.1% TFA) at a flow rate of 4 mL/min in 45 min to obtain stolonine C (**3**, 0.3 mg, 0.0021% dry wt in total) in fraction 33 and stolonine B (**2**, 1.2 mg, 0.0063% dry wt) in fractions 34–36.

Stolonine A (**1**): white, amorphous solid; UV (MeOH) λ_{max} (log ε) 210 (3.8), 252 (3.5) and 325 (3.3) nm; IR (film) ν_{max} 3307, 1681, 1205, 1049 and 802 cm^{-1}; ^{1}H (600 MHz, DMSO-d_6) and ^{13}C (150 MHz, DMSO-d_6) NMR data are summarized in Table 1; (−)-HRESIMS m/z 295.0390 $[M-H]^-$ (calcd for $[C_{12}H_{11}N_2O_5S]^-$, 295.0394, Δ −1.4 ppm).

Stolonine B (**2**): white, amorphous solid; UV (MeOH) λ_{max} (log ε) 210 (3.8) and 240 (3.9) nm; IR (film) ν_{max} 3386, 1684, 1204 and 1066 cm^{-1}; ^{1}H (600 MHz, DMSO-d_6) and ^{13}C (150 MHz,

DMSO-d_6) NMR data are summarized in Table 3; (−)-HRESIMS m/z 279.0441 [M − H]$^-$ (calcd for [$C_{12}H_{11}N_2O_4S$]$^-$, 279.0445, Δ −1.4 ppm).

Stolonine C (**3**): white, amorphous solid; UV (MeOH) λ_{max} (log ε) 210 (4.1) and 272 (3.8) nm; IR (film) ν_{max} 3418, 1682, 1197 and 1034 cm^{-1}; ^{1}H (600 MHz, DMSO-d_6) and ^{13}C (150 MHz, DMSO-d_6) NMR data are summarized in Table 4; (−)-HRESIMS m/z 318.0550 [M − H]$^-$ (calcd for [$C_{14}H_{12}N_3O_4S$]$^-$, 318.0554, Δ −1.3 ppm).

Synthetic stolonine A (**1**): To a solution of taurine (12 mg, 0.096 mmol) in dry DMF (1 mL) was added HOBt (26 mg, 0.193 mmol) and the reaction mixture was stirred for 15 min at rt. The reaction mixture was then cooled to 0 °C, EDCI (37 mg, 0.193 mmol) was added and continued stirring for 30 min at 0 °C. To this mixture was then added 3-indoleglyoxylic acid (**6**, 18 mg, 0.095 mmol) and the mixture was stirred for 21 h at rt. The crude product was concentrated *in vacuo* and separated by RP-HPLC (MeOH, H_2O, 0.1% TFA) to obtain the synthetic stolonine A (18 mg, 64%); IR (film) ν_{max} 3371, 1681, 1205, 1047, 802 and 749 cm^{-1}; ^{1}H (600 MHz, DMSO-d_6) and ^{13}C (150 MHz, DMSO-d_6) NMR data are summarized in Table 5; (−)-HRESIMS m/z 295.0391 [M − H]$^-$ (calcd for [$C_{12}H_{11}N_2O_5S$]$^-$, 295.0394, Δ −1.0 ppm).

Quinoline-2-carboxylic acid (**8**): To a solution of *o*-nitrobenzaldehyde (**7**, 302 mg, 2 mmol) in ethanol (5 mL) was added iron powder (504 mg, 9 mmol), followed by 0.1 N HCl (2 mL, 0.2 mmol) and the resulting mixture was vigorously stirred under reflux for 45 min. Methyl pyruvate (200 μL, 2 mmol) and powder KOH (135 mg, 2.4 mmol) were added slowly. The reaction mixture was stirred under reflux for 90 min and then cooled to rt. The crude product was purified by RP-HPLC (MeOH, H_2O, 0.1% TFA) to yield **8** (190 mg, 55% in two steps); ^{1}H NMR (500 MHz, DMSO-d_6) δ 8.56 (1H, d, J = 8.5 Hz), 8.16 (1H, d, J = 8.0 Hz), 8.11 (1H, d, J = 8.5 Hz), 8.09 (1H, d, J = 8.0 Hz), 7.88 (1H, t, J = 8.0 and 7.5 Hz) and 7.74 (1H, t, J = 8.0 and 7.5 Hz); ^{13}C NMR (125 MHz, DMSO-d_6) δ 166.2 (COOH), 148.5 (C), 146.6 (C), 137.6 (CH), 130.5 (CH), 129.5 (CH), 128.7 (C), 128.5 (CH), 127.9 (CH) and 120.6 (CH). (+)-LRESIMS m/z 174.

Synthetic stolonine B (**2**): To a solution of taurine (13 mg, 0.104 mmol) in dry DMF (1 mL) was added HOBt (28 mg, 0.207 mmol) and the reaction mixture was stirred for 15 min at rt. The reaction mixture was then cooled to 0 °C, EDCI (40 mg, 0.209 mmol) was added and continued stirring for 30 min at 0 °C. To this mixture was then added compound **8** (18 mg, 0.104 mmol) and the mixture was stirred for 48 h at rt. The pure synthetic stolonine B was purified by RP-HPLC (MeOH, H_2O, 0.1% TFA) to obtain 21.8 mg (75% yield); IR (film) ν_{max} 3383, 1677, 1201 and 1064 cm^{-1}; ^{1}H (600 MHz, DMSO-d_6) and ^{13}C (150 MHz, DMSO-d_6) NMR data are summarized in Table 5; (−)-HRESIMS m/z 279.0446 [M − H]$^-$ (calcd for [$C_{12}H_{11}N_2O_4S$]$^-$, 279.0445, Δ 0.4 ppm).

β-carboline-3-carboxylic acid (**10**): Formaldehyde (37%, 2 mL) was added to L-tryptophan methyl ester hydrochloride (**9**) (2.54 g, 10 mmol) in aqueous MeOH (10 mL, MeOH-H_2O (10:1)). The resulting mixture was stirred at rt for 16 h. The reaction mixture was evaporated to dryness *in vacuo* and oxidized by activated MnO_2 (2.5 g, 28.7 mmol) in benzene under reflux for 5 h. The hot solution was filtered through a bed of C_{18} to remove the MnO_2 and the filter cake was washed with hot benzene. The crude product was suspended in a mixture of aq. NaOH 20% and MeOH (ratio 1:4) and heated to reflux for 45 min. The reaction was cooled to rt, evaporated to dryness *in vacuo* and then loaded onto RP-HPLC (MeOH, H_2O, 0.1% TFA) yielding **10** (215 mg, 10% in three steps). ^{1}H NMR (600 MHz, DMSO-d_6) δ 12.07 (1H, s), 8.98 (1H, s), 8.92 (1H, s), 8.39 (1H, d, J = 8.4 Hz), 7.67 (1H, d, J = 8.4 Hz), 7.60 (1H, t, J = 7.2, 7.8 Hz), 7.31 (1H, t, J = 7.2, 7.8 Hz); ^{13}C NMR (150 MHz, DMSO-d_6) δ 166.8 (COOH), 141.1 (C), 137.4 (2xC), 133.1 (CH), 128.7 (CH), 127.8 (C), 122.2 (CH), 120.9 (C), 120.1 (CH), 117.2 (CH), 112.3 (CH). (+)-LRESIMS m/z 213.

Synthetic stolonine C (**3**): To a solution of taurine (5 mg, 0.040 mmol) in dry DMF (1 mL) was added HOBt (13.5 mg, 0.1 mmol) and the reaction mixture was stirred for 15 min at rt. The reaction mixture was then cooled to 0 °C, EDCI (19 mg, 0.099 mmol) was added and continued stirring for 30 min at 0 °C. To this mixture was then added **10** (8 mg, 0.038 mmol) and the mixture was stirred for 16 h at rt. The crude product was concentrated *in vacuo* and separated by RP-HPLC (MeOH, H_2O,

0.1% TFA) to obtain the synthetic stolonine C (4.8 mg, 40%); IR (film) ν_{max} 3419, 1683, 1198 and 1034 cm^{-1}; ^1H (600 MHz, DMSO-d_6) and ^{13}C (150 MHz, DMSO-d_6) NMR data are summarized in Table 5; (−)-HRESIMS m/z 318.0556 $[M-H]^-$ (calcd for $[C_{14}H_{12}N_3O_4S]^-$, 318.0554, Δ 0.6 ppm).

3.4. Computational Details

Molecular mechanics calculations were performed using Macromodel [40] interfaced to the Maestro program [41]. All conformational searches used the MMFFs force field. Twenty-one conformers of **1-I** and six conformers of **1-II** within a relative energy of 2 kcal/mol were found. The geometries of these conformers were subsequently optimized at DFT level with the B3LYP functional and 6-31G(d) basis set using Jaguar [42]. Single point calculations in DMSO with the mPW1PW91 functional and the same basis set were employed using Jaguar [42] to provide the shielding constant of carbon and proton nuclei. Meanwhile, the same procedure was applied on tetramethylsilane (TMS). Final ^1H and ^{13}C chemical shifts were obtained as the results of the Boltzmann weighted average. The theoretical chemical shifts were calculated according to a below equation.

$$\delta^x_{calc} = \sigma_{TMS} - \sigma^x \quad (1)$$

where δ^x_{calc} is the calculated shift for nucleus x (in ppm); σ^x is the shielding constant for nucleus x; σ_{TMS} is the shielding constant for the carbon in TMS σ_{TMS} = 194.6867 ppm and for the proton in TMS σ_{TMS} = 32.0845 ppm.

Statistical parameters were used to quantify the agreement between experimental and calculated data:

- The slope (a), the intercept (b) and the correlation coefficient (R^2) were determined from a plot of δ_{calc} against δ_{exp} for each particular compound.
- Systematic errors during the shift calculation were removed by empirical scaling according to $\delta_{scaled} = (\delta_{calc} - b)/a$
- The corrected mean absolute error (CMAE) was defined as $\sum_{i=1}^{n} |\delta_{scaled} - \delta_{exp}|/n$
- DP4 parameter was calculated by using the online applet [43].

3.5. Cytotoxicity Assay

Human prostate adenocarcinoma cells (PC3) and human neonatal foreskin fibroblast (noncancer cells, NFF) were grown in media RPMI-1640 (Life Technologies, Grand Island, NY, USA) supplemented with 10% foetal bovine serum (FBS) (Life Technologies, Grand Island, NY, USA). Cells were grown under 5% CO_2 in a humidified environment at 37 °C. Fifty microliters of media containing 500 cells were added to a 384 well microtiter plate (Perkin Elmer, Shelton, CT, USA, part number: 6,007,660) containing 0.2 μL of a compound. Final compound concentrations tested were 20, 6.5, 2, 0.65, 0.2, 0.065, 0.020 and 0.0065 μM (final DMSO concentration of 0.4%). Each concentration in media was tested in triplicate and in two independent experiments. Cells and compounds were then incubated in 72 h at 37 °C, 5% CO_2 and 80% humidity. Cell proliferation was measured with the addition of 10 μL of a 60% Alamar blue (Invitrogen, Carlsbad, CA, USA) solution in media to each well of the microtiter plate to give a final concentration of 10% Alamar blue. The plates were incubated at 37 °C, 5% CO_2 and 80% humidity within 24 h. The fluorescence of each well was read at excitation 535 nm and emission 590 nm on the Perkin Elmer EnVision Multilabel Reader 2104. Eight-point concentration response curves were then analyzed using non-linear regression and IC_{50} values determined by using GraphPad Prism 5 (GraphPad Software Inc., La Jolla, CA, USA). Paclitaxel and doxorubicin were used during each screening as positive control compounds.

3.6. Immunofluorescence Staining

Cells (2000 cells/well) were allowed to seed in a 96-well plate (CellCarrier, Perkin Elmer, Shelton, CT, USA, part number: 6,005,558) containing 0.4 μL of a compound at room temperature for 30 min and then placed under 5% CO_2 in a humidified environment at 37 °C. After 72 h incubation, 100 μL of a solution containing 1/1000 Hoechst 33,342 (Molecular Probes, Invitrogen, Carlsbad, CA, USA), 1 μM MitoTracker Deep Red (Molecular Probes, Invitrogen, Carlsbad, CA, USA) and 1/1000 CellMask Plasma Membrane (Molecular Probes, Invitrogen, Carlsbad, CA, USA) were added to each well and incubated for 30 min at 37 °C. Stained cells were washed once with PBS to remove excess stains and then replaced with 100 μL of PBS before being imaged.

3.7. Automated Microscopy and Image Analysis

Plates were imaged with an Operetta high-content wide-field fluorescence imaging system, coupled to Harmony software (Perkin Elmer, Shelton, CT, USA). Wells in a 96-well plate were captured at 25 locations per well at 20× magnification at three wavelengths (350 nm: Hoechst 33,342; 554 nm: CellMask Plasma Membrane; 644 nm: MitoTracker Deep Red). The three images were combined and analyzed using the Harmony software. The analysis protocol involved in the following steps: (1) each cell nucleus was identified using Hoechst stain; (2) the cell cytoplasm as defined from CellMask fluorescence; (3) cells that overlapped the border of the image were excluded from the analysis. Each concentration was repeated in at least two separated experiments. To obviate observer bias, the image analysis was automated using the same parameters for every image.

4. Conclusions

Contributing to the chemical study on the underexplored marine tunicate *Cnemidocarpa stolonifera*, three new alkaloids stolonines A–C (**1–3**) belonging to the taurine amide structure class were identified. Structures of these compounds were determined by NMR spectroscopy and confirmed by synthetic methods. Stolonines A–C (**1–3**) represent the 48–50th naturally occurring taurine amide compounds. However, this is the first time that the conjugates of taurine with 3-indoleglyoxylic acid, quinoline-2-carboxylic acid and β-carboline-3-carboxylic acid have been reported. Although compounds **1–3** displayed no cytotoxicity against the prostate cancer PC3 cells at the concentration of 20 μM, an immunofluorescence assay on PC3 cells revealed that compounds **1** and **3** increased cell size, induced mitochondrial texture elongation and affected the PC3 cell death via apoptotic pathway. Further investigation would be necessary to understand their mechanism of action on PC3 cells.

Supplementary Materials: IR, 1D and 2D NMR spectra of stolonines A–C (**1–3**) and other synthetic compounds (**8** and **10**); and calculated ^{13}C and ^{1}H NMR chemical shifts for each conformer of compounds **1-I** and **1-II**.

Acknowledgments: One of the authors (T.D.T.) acknowledges Griffith University for the provision of the "Griffith University International Postgraduate Research Scholarship and Griffith University Postgraduate Research Scholarship". We thank H. T. Vu at Eskitis Institute, Griffith University for acquiring the HRESIMS measurement and G. Pierens at Center for Advanced Imaging, University of Queensland for acquiring the 900 MHz NMR measurement. We acknowledge the Australian Research Council for support toward NMR and MS equipment (ARC LE0668477 and ARC LE0237908) and funding (ARC Discovery DP130102400).

Author Contributions: Ronald J. Quinn conceived and designed the research. Ronald J. Quinn and Ngoc B. Pham supervised the chemical experiments, structure elucidation, DFT calculations, synthesis and biological experiments. Trong D. Tran performed the natural product isolation, structural identification, DFT calculations, synthesis, cytotoxicity assays, immunofluorescence staining and cell imaging. John N. A. Hooper and Merrick Ekins collected and identified the tunicate samples. Trong D. Tran, Ngoc B. Pham and Ronald J. Quinn interpreted the results and wrote the manuscript.

Conflicts of Interest: The authors declare no conflict of interest.

References

1. Dias, D.A.; Urban, S.; Roessner, U. A historical overview of natural products in drug discovery. *Metabolites* **2012**, *2*, 303–336. [CrossRef] [PubMed]
2. Bergmann, W.; Feeney, R.J. The isolation of a new thymine pentoside from sponges. *J. Am. Chem. Soc.* **1950**, *72*, 2809–2810. [CrossRef]
3. Bergmann, W.; Feeney, R.J. Contributions to the study of marine products. XXXII. The nucleosides of sponges. I. *J. Org. Chem.* **1951**, *16*, 981–987. [CrossRef]
4. Hu, G.P.; Yuan, J.; Sun, L.; She, Z.G.; Wu, J.H.; Lan, X.J.; Zhu, X.; Lin, Y.C.; Chen, S.P. Statistical research on marine natural products based on data obtained between 1985 and 2008. *Mar. Drugs* **2011**, *9*, 514–525. [CrossRef] [PubMed]
5. Mehbub, M.F.; Lei, J.; Franco, C.; Zhang, W. Marine sponge derived natural products between 2001 and 2010: Trends and opportunities for discovery of bioactives. *Mar. Drugs* **2014**, *12*, 4539–4577. [CrossRef] [PubMed]
6. Leal, M.C.; Puga, J.; Serodio, J.; Gomes, N.C.M.; Calado, R. Trends in the discovery of new marine natural products from invertebrates over the last two decades—Where and what are we bioprospecting? *PLoS ONE* **2012**, *7*, e30580. [CrossRef] [PubMed]
7. Camp, D.; Newman, S.; Pham, N.B.; Quinn, R.J. Nature bank and the queensland compound library: Unique international resources at the eskitis institute for drug discovery. *Comb. Chem. High Throughput Screen.* **2014**, *17*, 201–209. [CrossRef] [PubMed]
8. Quinn, R.J.; Carroll, A.R.; Pham, N.B.; Baron, P.; Palframan, M.E.; Suraweera, L.; Pierens, G.K.; Muresan, S. Developing a drug-like natural product library. *J. Nat. Prod.* **2008**, *71*, 464–468. [CrossRef] [PubMed]
9. Tran, T.D.; Pham, N.B.; Fechner, G.; Quinn, R.J. Chemical investigation of drug-like compounds from the australian tree, *Neolitsea dealbata*. *Bioorg. Med. Chem. Lett.* **2010**, *20*, 5859–5863. [CrossRef] [PubMed]
10. Camp, D.; Davis, R.A.; Campitelli, M.; Ebdon, J.; Quinn, R.J. Drug-like properties: Guiding principles for the design of natural product libraries. *J. Nat. Prod.* **2012**, *75*, 72–81. [CrossRef] [PubMed]
11. Tran, T.D.; Pham, N.B.; Quinn, R.J. Structure determination of pentacyclic pyridoacridine alkaloids from the australian marine organisms *Ancorina geodides* and *Cnemidocarpa stolonifera*. *Eur. J. Org. Chem.* **2014**, *2014*, 4805–4816. [CrossRef]
12. Bittner, S.; Win, T.; Gupta, R. Gamma-L-glutamyltaurine. *Amino Acids* **2005**, *28*, 343–356. [CrossRef] [PubMed]
13. Chung, M.C.; Malatesta, P.; Bosquesi, P.L.; Yamasaki, P.R.; Santos, J.L.D.; Vizioli, E.O. Advances in drug design based on the amino acid approach: Taurine analogues for the treatment of CNS diseases. *Pharmaceuticals* **2012**, *5*, 1128–1146. [CrossRef] [PubMed]
14. Carbone, M.; Núñez-Pons, L.; Ciavatta, M.L.; Castelluccio, F.; Avila, C.; Gavagnin, M. Occurrence of a taurine derivative in an Antarctic glass sponge. *Nat. Prod. Commun.* **2014**, *9*, 469–470. [PubMed]
15. *Dictionary of Natural Products 23.2 Online*; Taylor & Francis Group: FL, USA, 2015.
16. Pretsch, E.; Buhlmann, P.; Badertscher, M. *Structure Determination of Organic Compounds*; Springer: Berlin, Germany, 2009.
17. Hosoya, T.; Hirokawa, T.; Takagi, M.; Shin-ya, K. Trichostatin analogues JBIR-109, JBIR-110, and JBIR-111 from the marine sponge-derived *Streptomyces* sp. RM72. *J. Nat. Prod.* **2012**, *75*, 285–289. [CrossRef] [PubMed]
18. Gupta, P.; Sharma, U.; Schulz, T.C.; McLean, A.B.; Robins, A.J.; West, L.M. Bicyclic C21 terpenoids from the marine sponge *Clathria compressa*. *J. Nat. Prod.* **2012**, *75*, 1223–1227. [CrossRef] [PubMed]
19. Bi, D.; Chai, X.Y.; Song, Y.L.; Lei, Y.; Tu, P.F. Novel bile acids from bear bile powder and bile of geese. *Chem. Pharm. Bull.* **2009**, *57*, 528–531. [CrossRef] [PubMed]
20. Smith, S.G.; Goodman, J.M. Assigning stereochemistry to single diastereoisomers by GIAO NMR calculation: The DP4 probability. *J. Am. Chem. Soc.* **2010**, *132*, 12946–12959. [CrossRef] [PubMed]
21. Micco, S.D.; Zampella, A.; D'Auria, M.V.; Festa, C.; Marino, S.D.; Riccio, R.; Butts, C.P.; Bifulco, G. Plakilactones G and H from a marine sponge. Stereochemical determination of highly flexible systems by quantitative NMR-derived interproton distances combined with quantum mechanical calculations of ^{13}C chemical shifts. *Beilstein J. Org. Chem.* **2013**, *9*, 2940–2949. [CrossRef] [PubMed]
22. Brown, S.G.; Jansma, M.J.; Hoye, T.R. Case study of empirical and computational chemical shift analyses: Reassignment of the relative configuration of phomopsichalasin to that of diaporthichalasin. *J. Nat. Prod.* **2012**, *75*, 1326–1331. [CrossRef] [PubMed]

23. Wyche, T.P.; Hou, Y.; Rivera, E.V.; Braun, D.; Bugni, T.S. Peptidolipins B–F, antibacterial lipopeptides from an ascidian-derived *Nocardia* sp. *J. Nat. Prod.* **2012**, *75*, 735–740. [CrossRef] [PubMed]
24. Wyche, T.P.; Hou, Y.; Braun, D.; Cohen, H.C.; Xiong, M.P.; Bugni, T.S. First natural analogs of the cytotoxic thiodepsipeptide thiocoraline A from a marine *Verrucosispora* sp. *J. Org. Chem.* **2011**, *76*, 6542–6547. [CrossRef] [PubMed]
25. Paterson, I.; Dalby, S.M.; Roberts, J.C.; Naylor, G.J.; Guzman, E.A.; Isbrucker, R.; Pitts, T.P.; Linley, P.; Divlianska, D.; Reed, J.K.; *et al.* Leiodermatolide, a potent antimitotic macrolide from the marine sponge *Leiodermatium* sp. *Angew. Chem. Int. Ed.* **2011**, *50*, 3219–3223. [CrossRef] [PubMed]
26. Ienaga, K.; Higashiura, K.; Toyomaki, Y.; Matsuura, H.; Kimura, H. Simple peptide. II. Syntheses and properties of taurine dipeptides containing neutral α-amino acid. *Chem. Pharm. Bull.* **1988**, *36*, 70–77. [CrossRef] [PubMed]
27. Silverstein, R.M.; Webster, F.X.; Kiemle, D. *Spectrometric Identification of Organic Compounds*, 7th ed.; John Wiley & Son: Danvers, MA, USA, 2005.
28. Li, A.H.; Ahmed, E.; Chen, X.; Cox, M.; Crew, A.P.; Dong, H.Q.; Jin, M.; Ma, L.; Panicker, B.; Siu, K.W.; *et al.* A highly effective one-pot synthesis of quinolines from *o*-nitroarylcarbaldehydes. *Org. Biomol. Chem.* **2007**, *5*, 61–64. [CrossRef] [PubMed]
29. Chaniyara, R.; Tala, S.; Chen, C.W.; Zang, X.; Kakadiya, R.; Lin, L.F.; Chen, C.H.; Chien, S.I.; Chou, T.C.; Tsai, T.H.; *et al.* Novel antitumor indolizino[6,7-b]indoles with multiple modes of action: DNA cross-linking and topoisomerase I and II inhibition. *J. Med. Chem.* **2013**, *56*, 1544–1563. [CrossRef] [PubMed]
30. Yin, W.; Majumder, S.; Clayton, T.; Petrou, S.; VanLinn, M.L.; Namjoshi, O.A.; Ma, C.; Cromer, B.A.; Roth, B.L.; Platt, D.M.; *et al.* Design, synthesis, and subtype selectivity of 3,6-disubstituted β-carbolines at Bz/GABA(A)ergic receptors. SAR and studies directed toward agents for treatment of alcohol abuse. *Bioorg. Med. Chem.* **2010**, *18*, 7548–7564. [CrossRef] [PubMed]
31. Dewick, P.M. *Medicinal Natural Products: A Biosynthetic Approach*, 3rd ed.; John Wiley & Sons: Chichester, UK, 2009.
32. Felnagle, E.A.; Jackson, E.E.; Chan, Y.A.; Podevels, A.M.; Berti, A.D.; McMahon, M.D.; Thomas, M.G. Nonribosomal peptide synthetases involved in the production of medically relevant natural products. *Mol. Pharm.* **2008**, *5*, 191–211. [CrossRef] [PubMed]
33. Strieker, M.; Tanovic, A.; Marahiel, M.A. Nonribosomal peptide synthetases: Structures and dynamics. *Curr. Opin. Struct. Biol.* **2010**, *20*, 234–240. [CrossRef] [PubMed]
34. Hunt, M.C.; Siponen, M.I.; Alexson, S.E.H. The emerging role of acyl-coa thioesterases and acyltransferases in regulating peroxisomal lipid metabolism. *Biochim. Biophys. Acta* **2012**, *1822*, 1397–1410. [CrossRef] [PubMed]
35. Farrell, E.K.; Merkler, D.J. Biosynthesis, degradation and pharmacological importance of the fatty acid amides. *Drug Discov. Today* **2008**, *13*, 558–568. [CrossRef] [PubMed]
36. Bottone, M.G.; Santin, G.; Aredia, F.; Bernocchi, G.; Scovassi, C.P.I. Morphological Features of Organelles during Apoptosis: An Overview. *Cells* **2013**, *2*, 294–305. [CrossRef] [PubMed]
37. Akter, R.; Hossain, M.Z.; Kleve, M.G.; Gealt, M.A. Wortmannin induces MCF-7 breast cancer cell death via the apoptotic pathway, involving chromatin condensation, generation of reactive oxygen species, and membrane blebbing. *Breast Cancer (Dove Med. Press)* **2012**, *4*, 103–113. [PubMed]
38. Häcker, G. The morphology of apoptosis. *Cell Tissue Res.* **2000**, *301*, 5–17. [CrossRef] [PubMed]
39. Eidet, J.R.; Pasovic, L.; Maria, R.; Jackson, C.J.; Utheim, T.P. Objective assessment of changes in nuclear morphology and cell distribution following induction of apoptosis. *Diagn. Pathol.* **2014**, *9*. [CrossRef] [PubMed]
40. Schrödinger, LCC. *MacroModel, Version 9.9*; Schrödinger, LCC: New York, NY, USA, 2012.
41. Schrödinger, LCC. *Maestro, Version 9.3.5*; Schrödinger, LCC: New York, NY, USA, 2012.
42. Schrödinger, LCC. *Jaguar, Version 8.0*; Schrödinger, LCC: New York, NY, USA, 2012.
43. Assignment of stereochemistry and structure using NMR and DP4. Available online: http://www-jmg.ch.cam.ac.uk/tools/nmr/DP4/ (accessed on 18 June 2014).

marine drugs

MDPI

Article

Structure Elucidation of New Acetylated Saponins, Lessoniosides A, B, C, D, and E, and Non-Acetylated Saponins, Lessoniosides F and G, from the Viscera of the Sea Cucumber *Holothuria lessoni*

Yadollah Bahrami [1,2,3,4,*] and Christopher M. M. Franco [1,2,3,*]

1 Medical Biotechnology, Flinders Medical Science and Technology, School of Medicine, Flinders University, Adelaide SA 5042, Australia; yadollah.bahrami@flinders.edu.au
2 Centre for Marine Bioproducts Development, Flinders University, Adelaide SA 5042, Australia
3 Australian Seafood Cooperative Research Centre, Mark Oliphant Building, Science Park, Adelaide SA 5042, Australia
4 Medical Biology Research Center, Kermanshah University of Medical Sciences, Kermanshah 6714415185, Iran
* Authors to whom correspondence should be addressed; ybahrami@mbrc.ac.ir (Y.B.); chris.franco@flinders.edu.au (C.M.M.F.); Tel.: +61-872-218-563 (Y.B.); +61-872-218-554 (C.M.M.F.); Fax: +61-872-218-555 (Y.B. & C.M.M.F.).

Academic Editor: Alejandro M. Mayer
Received: 8 August 2014; Accepted: 1 January 2015; Published: 16 January 2015

Abstract: Sea cucumbers produce numerous compounds with a wide range of chemical structural diversity. Among these, saponins are the most diverse and include sulfated, non-sulfated, acetylated and methylated congeners with different aglycone and sugar moieties. In this study, MALDI and ESI tandem mass spectrometry, in the positive ion mode, were used to elucidate the structure of new saponins extracted from the viscera of *H. lessoni*. Fragmentation of the aglycone provided structural information on the presence of the acetyl group. The presence of the *O*-acetyl group was confirmed by observing the mass transition of 60 u corresponding to the loss of a molecule of acetic acid. Ion fingerprints from the glycosidic cleavage provided information on the mass of the aglycone (core), and the sequence and type of monosaccharides that constitute the sugar moiety. The tandem mass spectra of the saponin precursor ions $[M + Na]^+$ provided a wealth of detailed structural information on the glycosidic bond cleavages. As a result, and in conjunction with existing literature, we characterized the structure of five new acetylated saponins, Lessoniosides A–E, along with two non-acetylated saponins Lessoniosides F and G at *m/z* 1477.7, which are promising candidates for future drug development. The presented strategy allows a rapid, reliable and complete analysis of native saponins.

Keywords: sea cucumber; viscera; saponins; mass spectrometry; MALDI; ESI; HPCPC; triterpene glycosides; structure elucidation; bioactive compounds; marine invertebrate; Echinodermata; holothurian

1. Introduction

Sea cucumbers belonging to the class *Holothuroidea* of the *Echinodermata* phylum are marine invertebrates that produce a range of compounds that have the potential to be used in agriculture, and as pharmaceuticals, nutraceuticals and cosmeceuticals [1,2].

Saponins are the most important characteristic and abundant secondary metabolites in this species [3]. Sea cucumber saponins exert a wide range of medicinal and pharmacological properties.

Saponins are also the main bioactive compounds in many plant drugs and folk medicines, especially in the Orient.

Although sea cucumber saponins share common saponin features, their aglycones, also called sapogenins or genins, are significantly different from those reported in the plant kingdom [1]. These amphipathic compounds generally possess a triterpene or steroid backbone or aglycone (hydrophilic, lipid-soluble) connected glycosidically to a saccharide moiety (hydrophilic, water-soluble) [3–5]. Saponins are also produced by other marine organisms including asteroids [6], which also belongs to the phylum *Echinodermata*, and sponges of the phylum *Porifera* [7]. Sea cucumbers saponins are usually triterpene glycosides (derived from lanostane) [3] while those from starfish are steroid glycosides [6]. The sugar moieties mainly consist of D-xylose (Xyl), D-quinovose (Qui), 3-*O*-methyl-D-glucose (MeGlc), 3-*O*-methyl-D-xylose (MeXyl) and D-glucose (Glc), and sometimes 3-*O*-methyl-D-quinovose, 3-*O*-methyl-D-glucuronic acid and 6-*O*-acetyl-D-glucose. In the oligosaccharide chain, the first monosaccharide unit is always a xylose, whereas 3-*O*-methylglucose and/or 3-*O*-methylxylose are always the terminal sugars. The presence of two quinovose residues in a carbohydrate moiety is unique for sea cucumber and starfish glycosides.

There are more than 700 triterpene glycosides in various species of sea cucumbers [3,5,8–17], which are classified into four main structural categories based on their aglycone moieties: three holostane types containing a (1) 3β-hydroxyholost-9(11)-ene aglycone skeleton; (2) a 3β-hydroxyholost-7-ene skeleton and (3) an aglycone moiety different to other two holostane type aglycones, and a nonholostane aglycone [5,12,17,18]. The majority of saponins belong to the holostane type group [3, 12,13,19]. Most sea cucumber saponins comprise of a lanostane-3β-ol type aglycone with a γ-18 (20)-lactone in the D-ring of tetracyclic triterpene (3β,20*S*-dihydroxy-5α-lanostano-18,20-lactone) [5], sometimes containing shortened side chains; the glycone contains up to six monosaccharide units covalently connected to C-3 of the aglycone.

In sea cucumbers, the sugar residue has only one branch [13], whereas plant saponins may contain one, two or three saccharide chains, with a few having an acyl group bound to the sugar moiety [20]. One of the most noteworthy characteristics of many of the saponins from marine organisms is the sulfation of aglycone or sugar moieties [1], and in sea cucumbers the sulfation of one or more of Xyl, Glc, MeGlc and Qui residues have been reported [3,11]. Most of them are mono-sulfated glycosides with few occurrences of di- and tri-sulfated glycosides [13,17]. Another structural feature that has been found only in this series of aglycones is the presence of an acetoxyl group at C-16 and/ or in the lateral side of the aglycone (C-22 or C-23 and/or C-25). The other structural feature is the presence of a 12α-hydroxy group in the aglycone unit of saponins in the genus *Holothuria*; however some contain two hydroxy groups at positions 12α and 17α of the holostanol skeleton. Several triterpene glycosides (such as Holothurinoside X, Fuscocinerosides B and Scabraside B) isolated from the sea cucumber *Holothuria lessoni* contain a carbonyl group in the lateral chain [3,12]. The majority of saponins from Aspidochirotida sea cucumbers contain the 9(11)-double bond in their aglycone moiety, but most of the glycosides isolated from *Holothuria* are $\Delta^{9,11}$-glycosides.

Recently, a series of unusual non-holostane triterpene glycoside have been reported from sea cucumbers, belonging to order *Dendrochirotida*, which have a shortened side chain, and no lactone function. So far, only nine non-holostane acetylated saponins including Kurilosides A and C, Psolusoside B, Frondoside C, Cucumariosides A_2-7, A_2-8, A_8, A_9 and Koreoside A have been reported from the class *Holothuroidea*.

Similarities in structure of saponin glycosides leads to difficulties in purification, and this vitiates the complete structure elucidation of these molecules (especially isomers). High Performance Centrifugal Partition Chromatography (HPCPC) is effective in separating polar compounds and was employed successfully in obtaining purified saponins in this study.

The viscera of an Australian sea cucumber *Holothuria lessoni* (golden sandfish) [21] was selected as a source of saponins because we hypothesized that the internal organs contain high levels of compounds as the viscera are expelled from the sea cucumber in order to repel other sea animals. In relation to internal organs, the saponin content of the cuvierian tubules of *Holothuria* were found to be higher than the body wall on a weight basis [22,23]. We have recently reported [3,12] new saponins within the viscera of *H. lessoni*, and in this paper we present five new acetylated saponins and two related new non-acetylated isomers identified from the viscera using mass spectrometry.

Nuclear magnetic resonance (NMR) spectroscopy can provide extensive structural information for saponins, however larger quantities of high-purity samples are generally needed. This is complicated with fractions if the NMR signals overlap, making their assignments more difficult. Moreover, the measurement of the absolute configuration of the sugar moieties of a saponin cannot be completely solved by NMR methods alone [24]. Matrix-assisted laser desorption/ionization time-of-flight mass spectrometry (MALDI-ToF/MS) and electrospray ionization mass spectrometry (ESI-MS) techniques have become the preferred techniques for analyses of saponins. Mass spectrometry provides a highly sensitive platform for the analyses of saponin structures by generating product ions by the cleavage of the glycosidic bond.

Several studies reported that individual species have specific saponin congeners. However some congeners are common among different species. Even if the diversity is great, saponins from closely related species still retain the same molecular motif [11,25] and this property of saponins can be utilized for their taxonomic classification. Because of their internal and external roles the molecular structure of these compounds was most likely to be conserved within the species.

Mass spectrometry has a long history in the structure elucidation of saponins in both negative and positive ion modes. It has been extensively used to determine the molecular weight and the structure of the native aglycones as well as the glycosidic linkages in the oligosaccharide chain without degradation of the glycosides. Knowledge of the chemical structure of compounds is very important to determine the specific correlation between the structure and their molecular and biological mechanism(s) of actions. We expect that the results of this project will transform the value of the viscera of sea cucumbers into sources of high value products, important to human health and industry.

2. Results and Discussion

We reported the isolation and purification of several saponins from the viscera of sea cucumber species, *H. lessoni*, using ethanolic extraction, followed by solvent partition, then HPCPC. The extraction and purification procedures and the mass spectrometry analyses were described in detail in our previous publications [3,12].

The appropriate HPCPC fractions were pooled, based on their similar Rf values when run on thin-layer chromatography (TLC), and concentrated to dryness. Sodium ions were introduced to the samples before conducting the MS analysis, ensuring all saponins observed in the positive ion mode were predominantly singly charged sodium adducts $[M + Na]^+$; triterpene glycosides have a high affinity to alkali cations. The prominence of $[M + Na]^+$ also facilitated the analysis of saponins in mixtures or fractions. The saponin profile of each HPCPC fraction was then revealed by MALDI MS and ESI-MS [3,12]. MS^2 analyses identified key diagnostic ions produced by cleavage of the glycosidic bond including oligosaccharide and monosaccharide fragments [3,12,26]. Other visible peaks and fragments detected corresponded to the loss of other neutral moieties such as CO_2, H_2O or CO_2 coupled with H_2O.

2.1. Structure Determination of Saponins by ESI-MS

ESI-MS^n is a very effective and powerful technique to distinguish isomeric saponins as they generate different MS^n fragmentation profiles [27,28]. All saponin ions perceived in the ESI-MS spectrum of the HPCPC fractions were also analyzed by ESI-MS^2 in the positive ion mode. Previous MS^2 studies on HPCPC fractions 12, 14, 15 [3], 17, 18, 20 and 22 [12] obtained from the butanolic extract of viscera of sea cucumber *H. lessoni* yielded a number of new saponins. This analysis of fraction 18 gave complex spectra representing several saponin classes, also confirmed the presence of saponins reported in the literature and identified new saponin congeners (Supplementary Figure S1, and Figure 1 of [12]).

Fifteen major peaks were detected which corresponded to several known triterpene compounds (as summarized in Table 1 of [12]), including Holothurinosides C/C_1, Desholothurin A_1 and Desholothurin A (synonymous with Nobiliside 2a), Holothurinoside J_1, Fuscocinerosides B/C or Scabraside A or 24-dehydroechinoside A and Holothurin E, Holothurin A, Holothurinosides E/E_1/O/P, Holothurinoside M, Holothurinosides A/A_1/R/R_1/S/Q, Holothurinoside N, Holothurinoside I and Holothurinoside K_1 in addition to several new saponins [3,12]. The spectrum displays one dominant peak at *m/z* 1477.7, which corresponds to unidentified (new) saponins, with elemental compositions of $C_{68}H_{110}O_{33}$, $C_{66}H_{102}O_{35}$ and $C_{66}H_{118}O_{34}$.

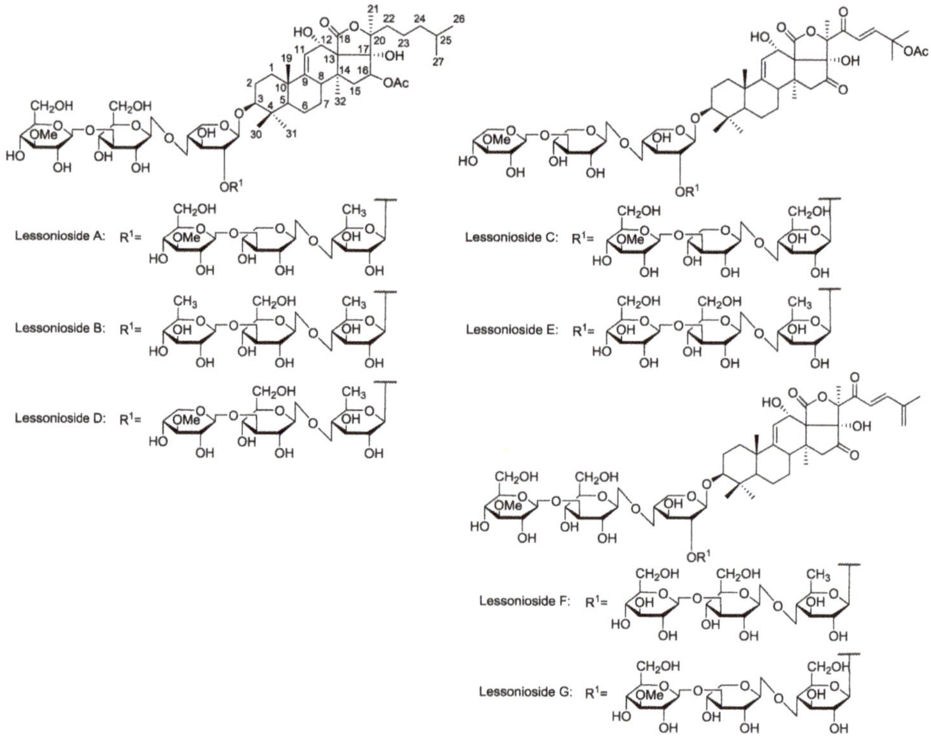

Figure 1. The structures of the new acetylated saponins in the viscera of *H. lessoni*, Lessoniosides (**A–E**) along with the non-acetylated Lessoniosides (**F–G**) compounds are described in this figure.

This analysis revealed that HPCPC Fraction 18 contains several saponin congeners showing that the absolute purification of the saponins was not possible within a single HPCPC run with these closely related compounds.

2.2. *Structure Identification of Saponins by MALDI-MS*

Similar to the ESI-MS, the MALDI MS of the isobutanol-enriched saponin extract obtained from the viscera of the *H. lessoni* revealed the presence of at least 75 saponin congeners, including 39 new sulfated, non-sulfated and acetylated triterpene glycosides, and 36 congeners which were previously reported in other holothurians [3].

To elucidate the chemical structure of saponins based on the MS^2 spectra, as described previously [3,12], precursor ions were selected, fragmented and fragmentation profiles built. The molecular structures of the saponins were determined by the identification of the mass transitions between the successive collision-induced fragmentation peaks on the basis of the accurate mass of the individual sugar components.

Based on the literature, MeGlc and MeXyl are always terminal sugars and Xyl is always the first sugar, which is bound to C-3 of the aglycone. Further, the exact mass of each sugar, such as MeGlc = 176 Da, Glc = 162 Da, Xyl = 132 Da, Qui = 146 Da, and the determination of the mass transitions between the peaks on the basis of the accurate mass of the individual sugar moieties, and mass and sequence of the key diagnostic peaks helped us build the sequence of these sugar moieties. Using this strategy the structure of seven new triterpene glycosides from *H. lessoni* with an *m/z* value of 1477.7 from HPCPC fraction 18 were characterized.

The chemical structures of the new acetylated saponins from the viscera of *H. lessoni* are illustrated in Figure 1. Lessoniosides A, B, C, D and E are the only published examples of glycosides from *H. lessoni* containing the side chain of the acetoxy group in their aglycone moieties. We now provide an account of the structure elucidation of these saponins using this approach.

MALDI-MS^2 Analysis of Saponins

Saponin ion peaks were further analyzed using MS^2 fingerprints generated with the collision-induced dissociation (CID) from their respective glycan structures. The techniques used are also able to distinguish the structural differences among the isomers following HPCPC separation. As a typical example, the MALDI-MS^2 fingerprints for the ion detected at *m/z* 1477.7 (triterpene glycoside) are shown in Figure 2. The schematic fragmentation of Lessonioside A as a representative is shown in Supplementary Figure S2. The fragmentation pattern of the sodiated compound at *m/z* 1477.7 in consecutive MS experiments is discussed in detail below for stepwise elucidation of the molecular structure of these compounds.

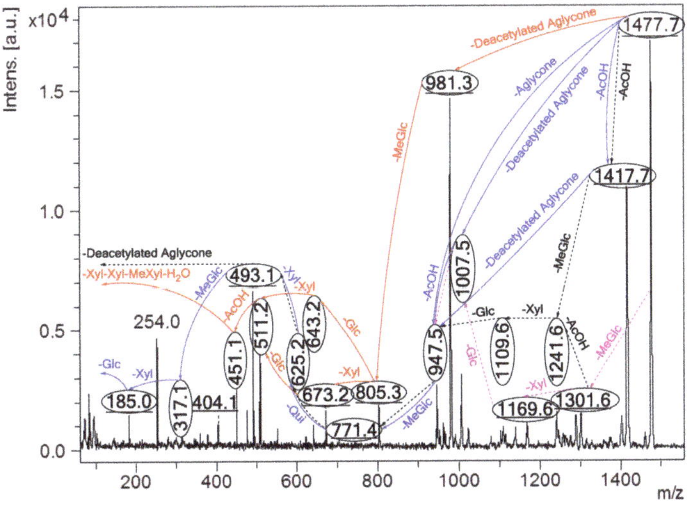

Figure 2. Positive tandem MALDI (matrix-assisted laser desorption/ionization) spectrum analyses of the precursor ion (saponin) detected at *m/z* 1477.7. The MS^2 fragmentation profile of the ion at *m/z* 1477.7. Figure shows the collision-induced fragmentation of parent ions at *m/z* 1477.7. The full and dotted arrows show the possible fragmentation pathways of this ion using CID (collision-induced dissociation). The blue arrows show the fragmentation of the isomeric congeners Lessonioside A where the red arrows indicate the decomposition patterns of Lessonioside C. These analyses revealed that this ion corresponds to isomeric compounds.

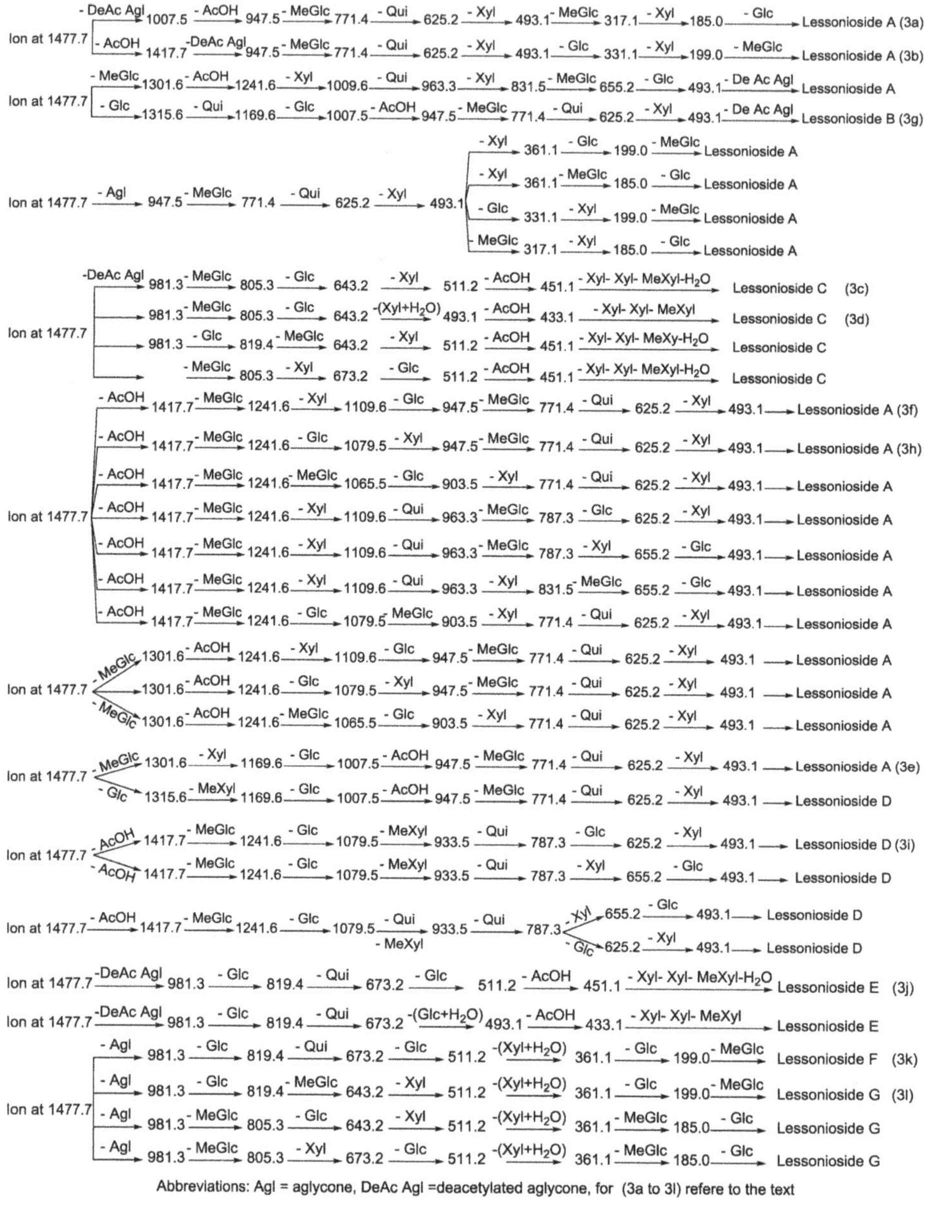

Figure 3. The schematic diagram of the proposed isomeric structures of the ion at *m/z* 1477.7. This figure indicates the comprehensive feasible fragmentation pathways of the isomeric acetylated, Lessoniosides (**A–E**), and non-acetylated, Lessoniosides (**F–G**), triterpene glycosides generated from the ion at *m/z* 1477.7.

CID activates three feasible independent fragmentation pathways of cationized parent ions shown in full and dotted arrows. First, as described in Figure 2, the consecutive losses of the deacetylated aglycone, acetic acid (AcOH), 3-*O*-methyl-D-glucose (MeGlc), D-quinovose (Qui), D-xylose (Xyl), MeGlc and Xyl residues (blue arrows) followed by D-glucose (Glc) yielded ion fragments at *m/z*

1007.5, 947.5, 771.4, 625.2, 493.1, 317.1 and 185.0 (Figure 3a), respectively, in one of the new isomers for which we propose the name Lessonioside A. The loss of aglycone (Agl) generated the ion at *m/z* 947, corresponding to the complete sugar moiety. The ion at *m/z* 493.1 corresponds to the diagnostic sugar reside $[MeGlc\text{-}Glc\text{-}Xyl + Na]^+$. Further, the sequential losses of Glc and Xyl units from this key diagnostic peak (*m/z* 493.1) generated ions at *m/z* 331.1 and 199.0 (Figure 3b).

With another isomer, the consecutive losses of the deacetylated aglycone, MeGlc, Glc, Xyl and AcOH followed by the hydrated three sugar units (red arrows) produced ions at *m/z* 981.3, 805.3, 643.2, 511.2 and 451.1, respectively, (Figure 3c) revealed the structure of a second new saponin, which we named Lessonioside C. Further, the consecutive losses of the deacetylated aglycone, MeGlc, Glc, Xyl (at a terminal position) and an acetyl group from the parent ion generated the fragment ions at *m/z* 981.3, 805.3, 643.2, 493.1 and 433.1, (Figure 3d) respectively, confirming the structure of Lessonioside C.

Secondly, the decomposition of the parent ion can also be triggered by the sequential loss of sugar moiety namely MeGlc, Xyl, Glc, AcOH, MeGlc, Qui and Xyl followed by the deacetylated aglycone residue which generated daughter ions at *m/z* 1301.6, 1169.6, 1007.5, 947.5, 771.4, 625.2, and 493.1, respectively (Figure 3e). This sequence of fragmentation confirms the structure of new saponin, Lessonioside A. In this case, the ions at *m/z* 493.1 correspond to the sodiated deacetylated aglycone moiety (*m/z* value of 470).

The third viable pathway is elicited by the initial loss of an acetoxy group. In the case of Lessonioside A this initial loss (−60) is followed by the sequential loss of the sugars (including the diagnostic MeGlc-Glc-Xyl) to yield the key diagnostic DeAc Agl ion (*m/z* 493.1) (Figure 3f). In addition the sequential losses of the MeGlc (317.1) and Xyl (*m/z* 185.0) followed by Glc further confirmed the structure of the new isomer, Lessonioside A.

As was observed with the MALDI-MS^2 this saponin possesses the common *m/z* 493.1 key signal diagnostic of both the sugar moiety $[MeGlc\text{-}Glc\text{-}Xyl + Na]^+$ and the DeAc Agl moiety $[C_{32}H_{50}O_6 - AcOH + Na]^+$. This is consistent with previous findings for the MS^2 of sea cucumber saponins [12]. The ion 493.1 is also observed in Lessonioside C, however, this is formed as a result of a loss of DeAc Agl and of the sugar moiety MeGlc-Glc-Xyl (511) and H_2O (493). The ion at 643 yields ions at 511 and 493 by the loss of Xyl and Xyl + H_2O, respectively. These ions are recognized as the key diagnostic fragments in triterpenoid saponins.

These MS^2 analyses using both MALDI and ESI modes allowed the establishment of connectivities of the sugar residues and thus permit the assignment of the peaks. For example, the MALDI-MS^2 of the parent ion showed fragments at *m/z* 1417.7 $[M + Na - AcOH]^+$ which suggested the presence of an acetyl moiety and the innate sugar component at *m/z* 947.5 $[M + Na - Agl]^+$, an observation that was confirmed by ESI- MS^2 in the positive ion mode. The MALDI mass spectrum showed evidence of the presence of the acetoxy group in the aglycone.

2.3. *Key Diagnostic Sugar Residues in the Sea Cucumber Saponins*

Characterization of common key fragments expedited the structure elucidation of new and reported saponins. Tandem mass spectrometry analysis of saponins showed the presence of several diagnostic key fragments corresponding to certain common structural element of saponins as summarized in Table 1. Here we report a new diagnostic key fragment at *m/z* 643 corresponding to the sodiated hydrated sugar residue MeGlc-Glc-Xyl-Xyl.

Table 1. Key diagnostic ions in the MS^2 of the holothurians saponins. It has been adapted from [12] and modified.

Diagnostic Ions in CID Spectra of Saponins $[M + Na]^+$				
	m/z Signals (Da)			
	493	507	643 or 625	639 or 657
Chemical signatures	MeGlc-Glc-Xyl + Na	MeGlc-Glc-Qui + Na	MeGlc-Glc-Xyl-Xyl + Na = 625 MeGlc-Glc-Xyl-Xyl + H_2O + Na = 643	MeGlc-Glc-Qui-Xyl + Na = 639 MeGlc-Glc-Qui-Xyl + H_2O + Na = 657

The structures of sugar components of saponins were established by the identification of these diagnostic ions produced by tandem mass spectrometry. Observing these oligosaccharide moieties (*m/z* 493 and/or 507 and/or 511 (493 + H_2O) and/or 523 and/or 643 and/or 657) simplified the characterization of the saponin structure.

2.4. Elucidation of the Saponin Structures by ESI-MS^2

ESI-MS^2 was carried out using CID, creating ion fragments from the precursor ions (Figure 4), and was applied to differentiate the structure of isomeric saponins as described by Song *et al.* [27]. The schematic fragmentation of Lessonioside A, as a representative, and the stepwise structure elucidation of the ion at *m/z* 1477.7 is shown in Figure 4 corroborates results from the MALDI-MS^2.

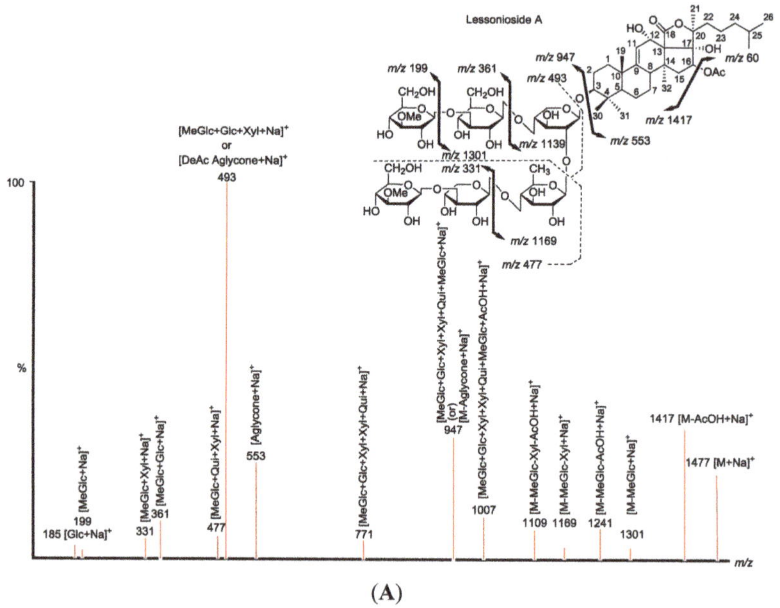

(A)

Figure 4. *Cont.*

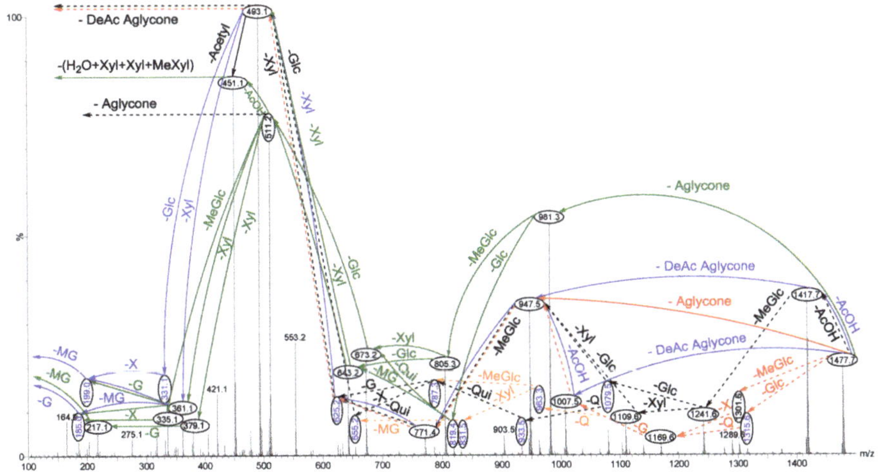

(B)

Figure 4. Positive ion mode ESI-MS^2 spectrum of acetylated saponins detected at *m/z* 1477.7 from Fraction 18. The schematic fragmentation of Lessonioside A as a representative (**A**), and the complete ESI-MS^2 fragmentation profile of the ion at *m/z* 1477.7 (**B**). Spectrum (**B**) shows the presence of two different aglycones in the isomeric saponins. Full and dotted arrows illustrate the three main feasible fragmentation pathways. The blue arrows show the decomposition of the isomeric congeners Lessoniosides A, B and D where the green arrows indicate the fragmentation patterns of Lessoniosides C, E, F and G. The ion at *m/z* 451.1 corresponds to the hydrated three sugar units [Xyl-Xyl-MeXyl + H_2O + Na].

2.4.1. ESI- MS^2 Analyses of Ion at *m/z* 1477.7

Tandem MS analyses revealed the presence of two different peaks with *m/z* value of 947.5 and 981.3, corresponding to the losses of different aglycone moieties with *m/z* values of 530 and 496, respectively, confirming the presence of chemical structural isomers. Further this MS^2 analysis also distinguished the presence of an acetoxy group in both isomer types.

Similar to sulfated compounds, after collisional activation, the parent ions are subjected to three independent dissociation pathways shown using full and dotted arrows (Figure 4). First, the consecutive losses of the deacetylated aglycone, acetoxy group, MeGlc, Qui, Xyl, Xyl and MeGlc residues (blue arrows) followed by Glc afford product ions as shown in Figure 4 confirmed the structure of Lessonioside A. Therefore, in this case, the ions at *m/z* 493.1 correspond to the sodiated key diagnostic sugar residue; [MeGlc-Glc-Xyl + Na]$^+$.

Secondly, the decomposition of the parent ion could also be triggered by the loss of sugar moieties followed by the deacetylated aglycone residue which generated daughter ions as shown in Figure 3e confirming once more the structure of Lessonioside A. It is clear that the ions at *m/z* 493.1 correspond to the sodiated deacetylated aglycone moiety (*m/z* value of 470). Alternatively, ions corresponding to the sequential losses of Glc, Qui, Glc, AcOH, MeGlc, Qui, and Xyl (red dotted arrows) were detected in Figure 3g indicating the presence of another isomer, Lessonioside B, which possesses two Qui units. The presence of two Qui in the carbohydrate chain of sea cucumber glycoside is a very rare characteristic.

Finally, the fragmentation of the parent ions can also be initiated with the loss of the acetoxy group. The consecutive losses of the acetic acid (AcOH) and the deacetylated aglycone unit followed by the sequential losses of the sugar moiety (Figure 3b) further confirmed the structure of Lessonioside A. Alternatively, the decomposition of the deacetylated saponins can be accomplished by the sequential losses of monosaccharides in the sugar chain, namely ion detected at 1417.7 [M − AcOH + Na]$^+$ (black dotted arrows, Figure 3h). In this case, the ions at 493.1 corresponds to the DeAc Agl moiety [M − sugar residue − AcOH + Na]$^+$. Alternatively, the sequential losses of AcOH and sugars from the parent ions (Figure 3i), afforded daughter ions that assisted in postulating the structure of another new isomer, Lessonioside D. The above evidence suggested that Lessonioside A possesses the same aglycone as Lessoniosides B and D, but differs in the hexasaccharide chain. The complete analyses can be seen in Supplementary Figure S3.

The MALDI-MS^2 and ESI-MS^2 analyses for all possible isomers were carried out in a similar manner as described above for Lessoniosides A, B, C and D. A comprehensive list of possible fragmentation patterns based on the MS^2 ions generated from the ion at *m/z* 1477.7 is shown in Figure 3.

The sugar moiety of Lessonioside A was found to be identical to those of Cladolosides C_1 and C_2 isolated from the sea cucumber *Cladolabes schmeltzii* [16], confirming the constituents of the hexasaccharide chain (Figures 1 and 3). The sugar component also had some similarity to those of Violaceuside B isolated from the sea cucumber *Pseudocolochirus violaceus* [29]. This group also stated the ions at *m/z* 625.2 and 493.1 corresponded to [MeGlc + Xyl + Glc + Xyl + Na]$^+$ and [MeGlc + Xyl + Glc + Na]$^+$, respectively, which confirmed our results. Yayli and associates [30], however, stated the ions at *m/z* 493 and 325, corresponding to [MeGlc-*O*-Xyl-*O*-Qui(*O*)-*O*]$^+$ and [MeGlc-*O*-Xyl]$^+$, respectively, which are under question. The structure of the aglycone moiety was also very similar to that of Holothurinoside Y [12], the difference being the addition of an acetoxy group at C-16. The assignments of the MS^2 signals associated with the aglycone moiety Lessoniosides A, B and D showed a close similarity to those reported for 16β-acetoxy-holosta-9-ene-3β,12α,17α-triol, the aglycone of Nobiliside C [*m/z* 715], *m/z* 656 [M − OAc + Na]$^+$, isolated from the sea cucumber *Holothuria nobilis* [31].

These saponin congeners identified from Fraction 18 are more conjugated with glycosides compared with the new saponins previously reported in this species [3,12]. Lessoniosides C, D and E possess the same terminal saccharide moiety (MeXyl), which is a rare structural feature among naturally occurring sea cucumber glycoside and has been infrequently reported.

2.4.2. Isomers that Generate the Deacetylated Aglycone at *m/z* 981.3

For other isomers, the loss of the deacetylated aglycone yields a large fragment at *m/z* 981.3. The alternative fragmentation patterns of the sugar residues for Lessoniosides C and E are described in Figure 3.

An interesting peculiarity of Lessonioside C and E is the presence of keto groups at both C-16 and C-22 positions, and 25β-*O*-Ac in the aglycone. This is the third example of the aglycone of sea cucumber glycosides bearing a ketone group at C-22 as Zhang *et al.* [32] and Liu *et al.* [33] stated the presence of a ketone group in Fuscocineroside A and Arguside D, respectively. The structure is characterized by the presence of an oligosaccharide chain composed of six units. The holostane-type aglycone features an endocyclic double bond at position C-9(11) and C-23 and a β-acetoxy group at C-25.

2.4.3. Non-Acetylated Isomeric Congeners

Based on the chemical evidence the structure of Lessoniosides F/G were defined as 16,22-diketo-holosta-9(11)-23(24)-25(27)-triene-3β,12α,17α-triol, which is shown in Figure 1. They are of the lanosterol type featuring the characteristic ring-D-fused γ-lactone (C=O) function and a Δ^9 double bond. The aglycone of Lessonioside F/G differs from E by the presence of a double bond at Δ^{25} and a loss of the AcO group at C-25 to form an exo double bond, Δ^{25}.

On fragmentation these isomers generate ions at 981.3 corresponding to the loss of aglycone. Subsequent losses of the sugar moieties are described in detail in Figure 3 (k and l) and Supplementary Figure S4 for Lessoniosides F and G. These non-acetylated Lessoniosides possess similar aglycones but different sugar moieties. It is notable that all three feasible independent fragmentation pathways might occur simultaneously which generated several different fragmentation sequences.

The molecular weights of the deacetylated aglycone moieties in some of these new saponins (Lessoniosides A, B and D) coincided with those reported for Philinopside B, from the sea cucumber *Pentacta quadrangularis* using ESI-MS by Zhang *et al.* [34], however, the structures are very different, because they are from a different family of sea cucumber, with ring closure of the C-20 side chain.

The cleavage of the *O*-acetyl group of the aglycone residue results in the loss of AcOH (60 Da). However, Song and co-workers [27] noted the neutral losses of CH_2O (30 Da) and $C_2H_4O_2$ (60 Da) in cross-ring reactions of the sugar residues. The cross-ring cleavage of the sugar also leads to the loss of $C_2H_4O_2$ (60 Da).

The losses of H_2O and CO_2 or their combination results from cleavage at the glycosidic linkages as noted by Waller and Yamasaki [2]. The losses of CO_2 (44 Da), H_2O (18 Da), AcOH (60 Da), Acetyl group (42 Da) and CH_2O (30 Da) were detected from the spectra which affords different product ions and several peaks were assigned to those molecules. For instance, the ion at *m/z* 1373.7 was generated by the loss of CO_2 from the deacetylated parent ions (*m/z* 1417.7), or the sequential losses of H_2O and acetyl molecule from the ions at *m/z* 511.2 generated ions at *m/z* 493.1 and 451.1, respectively. Further the ion at *m/z* 493.1 can be stemmed from the ion at *m/z* 553.2 (sodiated aglycone) by the loss of the acetoxy group. Additionally, the loss of CH_2O from the ion at *m/z* 451.1 yields the ion at *m/z* 421.1. However, Kelecom and coworkers [35], and Kitagawa and associates [36], stated the latter ion as an aglycone fragment. The complete analyses can be seen in the Supplementary Figure S3.

The MS^2 analyses of ions at *m/z* 1477.7 revealed a similar fingerprint profile with those reported for Holothurinosides X, Y and Z, in particular in the area of 100 to 600 Da where the signals were coincident with those of ion at *m/z* 1127.6, which show the intrinsic relationship between these saponin congeners [12].

Lessoniosides A, B, C, D and E are the only examples of glycosides from *H. lessoni* containing an acetoxy side chain in their aglycone moieties. Most of the glycosides isolated from sea cucumber *Holothuria* are $\Delta^{9,11}$- glycosides. In general, 3β-hydroxyholost-9(ll)-ene based aglycones were characterized in Holothurins isolated from animals of the order *Aspidochirota* [17].

2.5. The Structure of Aglycones

This analysis revealed the presence of at least seven different isomers with diverse aglycone and sugar components for the ion at *m/z* 1477.7. The glycosides differ in their aglycone structures or sugar moieties. The mass of the cationized aglycone and the deacetylated aglycone in Lessonioside C and E are 556 Da $[M - \text{sugar residue} + Na]^+$ and 496 $[M - AcOH - \text{sugar residue} + Na]^+$, respectively, which are consistent with the mass of the aglycone reported by Elyakov and co-workers [37]. Their MS analyses showed *m/z* 556 $[M]^+$, 541 $[M - CH_3]^+$ and 496 $[M - CH_3COO]^+$ for an aglycone moiety. Further, Rothberg and associates noted an aglycone with the same molecular weight having an acetoxy group at the C-23 from *Stichopus chloronotus* [38]. Analysis of the MS data for these isomers and comparison with those published for related saponin aglycones [3,12,31,39] shows that the aglycone part of Lessoniosides are a holostane skeleton featuring hydroxy groups at C-12 and C17. With other isomers, the mass of the cationized aglycone and the deacetylated aglycone was found to be 530 Da and 493 Da, respectively. Other prominent high mass ions *m/z* 1417 $[M - AcOH + Na]^+$ and 1241 $[M - AcOH - MeGlc + Na]^+$ or 1241 $[1301 - AcOH + Na]^+$ provide additional support for the acetate and lactone functions.

The aglycone structure of Lessoniosides C/E appears to be similar to that of Fuscocineroside A reported from the sea cucumber *Holothuria fuscocinerea* [32]. The lateral C-20 side chain of Lessoniosides C and E was found to be similar to Fuscocineroside A [32], and Arguside D [33]. However, they differed from Fuscocineroside A and Arguside D by the addition of a keto at C-16, a C-23 double bond and a 17-OH.

Three of these compounds, Lessoniosides A, B and D have identical holostane aglycones containing an 18(20)-lactone with a 9(11)-double bond and acetoxy group at C-16 and differ from each other in their sugar component. On the other hand, they differ from Lessoniosides C/E in the presence of an acetoxy group at the C-16 (*vs.* keto group in C/E) and absence of a C-22 keto group, a C-23 double bond and a C-25 acetoxy at the lateral chain.

These glycosides have holotoxinogenin, a genin containing 9(11)-double bond and 16-oxidized group in the aglycone. They possess two hydroxy groups at 12α and 17α positions that are characteristic for Aspidochirotid sea cucumber (the family *Holothuriidae*). This aglycone is common for glycosides from many different sea cucumbers [11].

Therefore, elucidation of the aglycone component of the saponins was performed by comparison with published data. Because the new identified compounds clearly have aglycone structures similar to that of other previously characterized compounds we can be confident that it is possible to elucidate the structure of these compounds based on MS analysis alone. However, NMR analysis will be required to confirm the structure of the aglycones and also to ascertain the stereochemistry and linkages of the sugar moieties. Whereas, in the case of a novel compound without any similar previously characterized components, detailed chemical analysis including the application of NMR would be required.

2.6. Acetylated Saponins

So far more than 700 triterpene glycosidic saponins have been reported from sea cucumber species of which more than 130 are acetylated saponin. The majority of these are of the holostane type. The known acetylated triterpene glycosides (saponins), isolated from sea cucumbers of the class *Holothuroidea*, possess an acetyl group (acetoxy) in their aglycone residues. In the *Holothuriidae* family, the acetoxy group is either located at C-16 of the aglycone core moiety such as in Arguside F [40] and Nobiliside C [31], or at the C-22, C23 or C-25 of the lateral chain, ie at C-25 of the Pervicosides A and D [40,41]. However, Cucumarioside A_1-2 is the only example of a triterpene glycoside containing an acetate group at C-6 (6-OAc) of the terminal glucose unit (sugar residue) 6-*O*-acetylglucose [42].

The majority of the acetylated compounds, such as Fuscocineroside A from the sea cucumber *H. fuscocinerea*, contain a sulfate group in their structures [32]. However, the presence of a sulfate group was not observed in these new acetylated saponins from *H. lessoni*.

Acetylated saponins are mainly reported in the family *Cucucmarridae*. However, the presence of acetylated saponins for the genus *Holothuria* is only reported for *H. lessoni* (this work), *H. pervicax*, *H. forskalii*, *H. nobilis*, *H. hilla*, *H. fuscocinerea*, *H. (Microthele) axiloga* and *H. pervicax* [17,31,32,40,41,43,44]. The majority of reported acetylated saponins possess only one acetoxy group in their structure, whereas saponins containing two *O*-acetic groups in their aglycone moieties have also been reported [16].

The presence of 12α and 17α–hydroxy, which are characteristic for glycosides from holothurians belonging to the family *Holothuriidae* (order *Aspidochirotida*), in glycosides of Dendrochirotids confirms parallel and relatively independent character of evolution of glycosides.

Observations from numerous studies confirm that the biological activity of saponins is influenced both by the aglycone and the sugar moiety. In other words there is a close relationship between the chemical structure of saponins and their biological activities. It has been reported that the presence of acetyl groups usually increases cytotoxic potency [45]. Therefore Lessoniosides seem to be potential candidates for anti-cancer drugs development.

3. Experimental Section

3.1. Sea Cucumber Sample

Twenty sea cucumber samples of *H. lessoni* [21], commonly known as Golden sandfish were collected off Lizard Island (latitude; 14°41′29.46″ S, longitude; 145°26′23.33″ E), Queensland, Australia on September 2010 [3,12]. The viscera (all internal organs) were separated from the body wall and kept separately in zip-lock plastic bags which were snap-frozen, then transferred to the laboratory and kept at −20 °C until use.

3.2. Extraction of Saponins

The saponins were extracted as described previously [3,12]. Briefly, the visceral masses were removed, freeze dried (VirTis, BenchTop K, New York, NY, USA) and pulverized to a fine powder using liquid nitrogen and a mortar and pestle. The pulverized viscera sample was extracted four times with 70% ethanol (EtOH) (400 mL) and filtered using Whatman filter paper (No. 1, Whatman Ltd., Maidstone, England, UK) at room temperature. The extract was concentrated under reduced pressure at 30 °C using a rotary evaporator (Büchi AG, Flawil, Switzerland) to remove the ethanol, and the residual sample was freeze-dried. The dried extract was dissolved in 400 mL of 90% aqueous methanol (MeOH), and partitioned against 400 mL of *n*-hexane twice. The water content of the hydromethanolic phase was then adjusted to 20% (v/v) and then to 40% (v/v) and the solutions partitioned against CH_2Cl_2 and $CHCl_3$, respectively. The hydromethanolic phase was concentrated and then freeze-dried. The dried powder was solubilized in 10 mL of MilliQ water (18.2 MΩ, Millipore, Bedford, MA, USA) in readiness for chromatographic purification.

3.3. Purification of the Extract

The aqueous extract was applied to an Amberlite® XAD-4 column (250 g XAD-4 resin 20–60 mesh; Sigma-Aldrich, MO, USA; 4 × 30 cm column) [3,12], washed extensively with water (1 L) and the saponins eluted sequentially with MeOH (450 mL), acetone (350 mL) and water (250 mL). The MeOH, acetone and water eluates were concentrated, dried, and redissolved in 5 mL of MilliQ water. Finally, the aqueous extract was partitioned with 5 mL isobutanol (v/v). The isobutanolic saponin-enriched fraction was either stored for subsequent mass spectrometry analyses or concentrated to dryness and the components of the extract were further purified by HPCPC. The profile of fractions was also monitored by TLC.

3.4. Thin Layer Chromatography (TLC)

Samples were dissolved in 90% or 50% aqueous MeOH and 10 μL were loaded onto silica gel 60 F_{254} aluminum sheets (Merck # 1.05554.0001, Darmstadt, Germany) and developed with the lower phase of $CHCl_3$:MeOH:H_2O (7:13:8) biphasic solvent system [3]. The profile of separated compounds on the TLC plate was visualized by UV light and by spraying with a 15% sulfuric acid in EtOH solution and heating for 15 min at 110 °C until maroon-dark purple spots developed.

3.5. High Performance Centrifugal Partition Chromatography (HPCPC or CPC)

The solvent system containing $CHCl_3$:MeOH:H_2O–0.1% HCO_2H (7:13:8) was mixed vigorously in a separating funnel and allowed to reach hydrostatic equilibration [3,12]. Following the separation of the two-immiscible phase solvent systems, both phases were degassed using a sonicator-degasser (Soniclean Pty Ltd. Adelaide, SA Australia). Then the rotor column of HPCPC™, CPC240 (Ever Seiko Corporation, Tokyo, Japan) was filled with the stationary phase (the aqueous upper phase) in the descending mode at a flow rate of 5 mL min^{-1} by Dual Pump model 214 (Tokyo, Japan), with a revolution speed of 300 rpm. The lower mobile phase was pumped in the descending mode at a flow rate of 1.2 mL min^{-1} with a rotation speed of 900 rpm within 2 h. One hundred and twenty milligrams of isobutanol-enriched saponins mixture was injected into the machine in the descending mode. The chromatogram was developed for 3 hours at 1.2 mL min^{-1} and 900 rpm using the Variable Wavelength UV-VIS Detector S-3702 (Soma optics, Ltd. Tokyo, Japan) and chart recorder (Ross Recorders, Model 202, Topac Inc. Cohasset, MA, USA). The fractions were collected in 3 mL tubes using a Fraction collector. At Fraction 54, the elution mode was switched to ascending mode and the aqueous upper phase was pumped at the same flow rate for 3 h to recover saponins. Fractions were monitored by TLC as described above. Monitoring of the fractions was necessary, as most of the saponins could not be detected by UV due to the lack of a chromophore structure. Fractions were concentrated with nitrogen gas.

3.6. Mass Spectrometry

The resultant HPCPC purified polar extracts were further analyzed by MALDI- and ESI-MS to elucidate and characterize the molecular structures of compounds.

3.6.1. MALDI MS

MALDI analysis was carried out using a Bruker Autoflex III Smartbeam (Bruker Daltonik, Bremen, Germany). All MALDI MS equipment, software and consumables were from Bruker Daltonics. The laser (355 nm) had a repetition rate of 200 Hz and operated in the positive reflectron ion mode for MS data over the mass range of 400 to 2200 Da under the control of the Flexcontrol and FlexAnalysis software (V 3.3 build 108). External calibration was performed using the sodium-attached ions from a Polyethylene Glycol of average molecular weight 1000. MS spectra were processed in FlexAnalysis (version 3.3, Bruker Daltonik, Bremen, Germany). MALDI MS^2 spectra were obtained using the LIFT mode of the Bruker Autoflex III with the aid of CID. The isolated ions were subjected to collision against argon in the collision cell to be fragmented, affording intense product ion signals. For MALDI a laser was used to provide both good signal levels and mass resolution with the laser energy for MS^2 analysis being generally 25% higher than for MS analysis.

The samples were spotted onto a MALDI stainless steel MPT Anchorchip TM 600/384 target plate. Alpha-cyano-4-hydroxycinnamic acid (CHCA) in acetone/iso-propanol in ratio of 2:1 (15 mg mL^{-1}) was used as a matrix to produce gas-phase ions. The matrix solution (1 μL) was placed onto the MALDI target plate and air-dried. Subsequently 1 μL of sample was added to the matrix crystals and air-dried [3,12]. Finally, 1 μL of NaI (Sigma-Aldrich # 383112, St Louis, MI, USA) solution (2 mg/mL in acetonitrile) was applied onto the sample spots. The samples were mixed on the probe surface and dried prior to analysis.

3.6.2. ESI MS

The ESI mass spectra were attained with a Waters Synapt HDMS (Waters, Manchester, UK). Mass spectra were acquired in the positive ion mode with a capillary voltage of 3.0 kV and a sampling cone voltage of 100 V.

The other conditions were as follows: extraction cone voltage, 4.0 V; ion source temperature, 80 °C; desolvation temperature, 350 °C; desolvation gas flow rate, 500 L h^{-1} [3,12]. Data acquisition was performed using a Waters MassLynx (V4.1, Waters Corporation, Milford, CT, USA). Positive ion mass spectra were acquired in the V resolution mode over a mass range of 100–2000 *m/z* using continuum mode acquisition. Mass calibration was performed by infusing sodium iodide solution (2 μg/μL, 1:1 (v/v) water:isopropanol). For accurate mass analysis a lock mass signal from the sodium attached molecular ion of Raffinose (*m/z* 527.1588) was used through the LockSpray source of the Synapt instrument.

MS^2 spectra were obtained by mass selection of the ion of interest using the quadrupole, fragmentation in the trap cell where argon was used as collision gas. Typical collision energy (Trap) was 50.0 V. Samples were infused at a flow rate of 5 μL/min, if dilution of the sample was required then acetonitrile was used [27]. Chemical structures were determined from fragmentation schemes calculated on tandem mass spectra and from the literature.

4. Conclusions

In recent years, there has been a great improvement in the number of MS applications. The tandem MS approach coupled with HPCPC separation revealed the structure of isomeric compounds containing different aglycones and/or sugar residues. Therefore, a creative and sensitive method has been developed for the structure elucidation of triterpene glycosides in sea cucumber and related products using HPCPC and MS. The result showed that this method is a rapid, accurate and reliable technique for the structure determination of triterpene glycosides in sea cucumber extracts.

This study proved the occurrence of both glycoside and cross-ring cleavages in the sugar moieties of sea cucumber saponins. The sequence of monosaccharide units and the presence of an acetoxy group, clearly reflected by the loss of 60 Da from the parent ions, were noted in five of the seven new saponins.

Tandem mass spectrometry data suggested that the most prominent ions generally stemmed from the losses of aglycones and/or the key diagnostic sugar moieties (*m/z* 493, 507, 511, 639, 643 and 625).

Our results also illustrate that some saponins are unique to the species, whilst others are common between multiple species. The MS analysis revealed that individual species possesses a unique saponin pattern in which some congeners are very specific to one species. This feature can be used for the taxonomic classification of sea cucumber species.

Characterization of some of these saponins were easier since their MS^2 spectra possessed the key diagnostic signal at *m/z* 493, corresponding to the oligosaccharide chain [MeGlc-Glc-Xyl + Na^+] in addition to the vital peak at *m/z* 643, corresponding to the oligosaccharide moiety [MeGlc-Glc-Xyl-Xyl-H_2O + Na^+]. Lessoniosides C, D and E contain 3-*O*-methylxylose as a terminal monosaccharide unit, which is a rare structural feature in sea cucumber triterpene glycosides.

The ion at *m/z* 1477.7 was identified as the major component of the glycoside fraction 18, containing holostane aglycones with 9(11)-double bond and 18(20)-lactone, characteristic for most of the known sea cucumber glycosides. The structures of these glycosides are quite different from those reported in this species. These substances contain aglycones with an oxidized position at C-16, (acetate group or keto group). Lessoniosides have the aglycone unit like that in Holothurinoside Y with an acetoxyl instead of hydrogen at position 16, but another aglycone moiety with the saturated side chain and with an acetoxyl (a 16β-acetate group) instead of a ketone at position 16.

Our results to date highlight the abundance of new saponins in the viscera indicating the viscera as a major source of these compounds with diverse structures. This paper is the first not only to deduce the structure of several new acetylated isomeric saponins, (Lessoniosides A–G) but also to present the structural diversity of triterpene glycoside congeners in the viscera of *H. lessoni*.

These new saponins (Lessoniosides A–G) have the potential to be consumed with applications as dietary supplements, food preservatives (because of their emulsifying and foaming properties), food additives and development of high value products for various industrial applications and as anti-cancer agents.

Our findings demonstrate that the marine world, in particular sea cucumbers, have much to offer human society in the way of nutraceuticals, pharmaceuticals, agrochemicals, cosmeceuticals, and research biochemicals.

Acknowledgments: We would like to express our sincerest thanks to the Australian SeaFood CRC for financially supporting this project and the Iranian Ministry of Health and Medical Education for their scholarship to YB, Ben Leahy and Tasmanian SeaFoods for supplying the sea cucumber samples. The authors gratefully acknowledge the technical assistance provided by Daniel Jardine and Jason Young at Flinders Analytical Laboratory, Elham Kakaei and Associate Prof. Michael Perkins at Flinders.

Author Contributions: Y.B. and C.F. designed the experiments. Y.B. carried out the experiments with guidance from C.F. Y.B. worked on chemical structure elucidation and both authors contributed in writing the manuscript.

Conflicts of Interest: The authors declare no conflict of interest.

References

1. Hostettmann, K.; Marston, A. *Saponins*; Cambridge University Press: Cambridge, UK, 1995.
2. Waller, G.R.; Yamasaki, K. *Saponins Used in Food and Agriculture*; Plenum Press: New York, NY, USA, 1996; Volume 405.
3. Bahrami, Y.; Zhang, W.; Franco, C. Discovery of novel saponins from the viscera of the sea cucumber *Holothuria lessoni*. *Mar. Drugs* **2014**, *12*, 2633–2667. [CrossRef] [PubMed]

4. Kerr, R.G.; Chen, Z. *In vivo* and *in vitro* biosynthesis of saponins in sea cucumbers. *J. Nat. Prod.* **1995**, *58*, 172–176. [CrossRef]
5. Kim, S.K.; Himaya, S.W. Triterpene glycosides from sea cucumbers and their biological activities. *Adv. Food Nutr. Res.* **2012**, *65*, 297–319. [PubMed]
6. Demeyer, M.; de Winter, J.; Caulier, G.; Eeckhaut, I.; Flammang, P.; Gerbaux, P. Molecular diversity and body distribution of saponins in the sea star *Asterias rubens* by mass spectrometry. *Comp. Biochem. Physiol. B* **2014**, *168*, 1–11. [CrossRef]
7. Regalado, E.L.; Tasdemir, D.; Kaiser, M.; Cachet, N.; Amade, P.; Thomas, O.P. Antiprotozoal steroidal saponins from the marine sponge *Pandaros acanthifolium*. *J. Nat. Prod.* **2010**, *73*, 1404–1410. [CrossRef] [PubMed]
8. Antonov, A.S.; Avilov, S.A.; Kalinovsky, A.I.; Anastyuk, S.D.; Dmitrenok, P.S.; Evtushenko, E.V.; Kalinin, V.I.; Smirnov, A.V.; Taboada, S.; Ballesteros, M.; *et al.* Triterpene glycosides from antarctic sea cucumbers 1. Structure of liouvillosides A_1, A_2, A_3, B_1, and B_2 from the sea cucumber *Staurocucumis liouvillei*: New procedure for separation of highly polar glycoside fractions and taxonomic revision. *J. Nat. Prod.* **2008**, *71*, 1677–1685. [CrossRef]
9. Van Dyck, S.; Gerbaux, P.; Flammang, P. Qualitative and quantitative saponin contents in five sea cucumbers from the Indian ocean. *Mar. Drugs* **2010**, *8*, 173–189. [CrossRef] [PubMed]
10. Kalinin, V.I.; Aminin, D.L.; Avilov, S.A.; Silchenko, A.S.; Stonik, V.A. Triterpene glycosides from sea cucucmbers (Holothuroidea, Echinodermata). Biological activities and functions. *Stud. Nat. Prod. Chem.* **2008**, *35*, 135–196.
11. Stonik, V.A.; Kalinin, V.I.; Avilov, S.A. Toxins from sea cucumbers (holothuroids): Chemical structures, properties, taxonomic distribution, biosynthesis and evolution. *J. Nat. Toxins* **1999**, *8*, 235–248. [PubMed]
12. Bahrami, Y.; Zhang, W.; Chataway, T.; Franco, C. Structural elucidation of novel saponins in the sea cucumber *Holothuria lessoni*. *Mar. Drugs* **2014**, *12*, 4439–4473. [CrossRef]
13. Kalinin, V.I.; Silchenko, A.S.; Avilov, S.A.; Stonik, V.A.; Smirnov, A.V. Sea cucumbers triterpene glycosides, the recent progress in structural elucidation and chemotaxonomy. *Phytochem. Rev.* **2005**, *4*, 221–236. [CrossRef]
14. Silchenko, A.S.; Kalinovsky, A.I.; Avilov, S.A.; Andryjaschenko, P.V.; Dmitrenok, P.S.; Kalinin, V.I.; Yurchenko, E.A.; Dautov, S.S. Structures of Violaceusosides C, D, E and G, sulfated triterpene glycosides from the sea cucumber *Pseudocolochirus violaceus* (Cucumariidae, Dendrochirotida). *Nat. Prod. Commun.* **2014**, *9*, 391–399. [PubMed]
15. Silchenko, A.S.; Kalinovsky, A.I.; Avilov, S.A.; Andryjaschenko, P.V.; Dmitrenok, P.S.; Martyyas, E.A.; Kalinin, V.I.; Jayasandhya, P.; Rajan, G.C.; Padmakumar, K.P. Structures and biological activities of Typicosides A_1, A_2, B_1, C_1 and C_2, triterpene glycosides from the sea cucumber *Actinocucumis typica*. *Nat. Prod. Commun.* **2013**, *8*, 301–310. [PubMed]
16. Silchenko, A.S.; Kalinovsky, A.I.; Avilov, S.A.; Andryjaschenko, P.V.; Dmitrenok, P.S.; Yurchenko, E.A.; Dolmatov, I.Y.; Kalinin, V.I.; Stonik, V.A. Structure and biological action of Cladolosides B_1, B_2, C, C_1, C_2 and D, six new triterpene glycosides from the sea cucumber *Cladolabes schmeltzii*. *Nat. Prod. Commun.* **2013**, *8*, 1527–1534. [PubMed]
17. Chludil, H.D.; Murray, A.P.; Seldes, A.M.; Maier, M.S. Biologically active triterpene glycosides from sea cucumbers (Holothuroidea, Echinodermata). *Stud. Nat. Prod. Chem.* **2003**, *28*, 587–615.
18. Avilov, S.A.; Kalinovsky, A.I.; Kalinin, V.I.; Stonik, V.A.; Riguera, R.; Jiménez, C. Koreoside A, a new nonholostane triterpene glycoside from the sea cucumber *Cucumaria koraiensis*. *J. Nat. Prod.* **1997**, *60*, 808–810. [CrossRef] [PubMed]
19. Zou, Z.R.; Yi, Y.H.; Wu, H.M.; Wu, J.H.; Liaw, C.C.; Lee, K.H. Intercedensides A–C, three new cytotoxic triterpene glycosides from the sea cucumber *Mensamaria intercedens* Lampert. *J. Nat. Prod.* **2003**, *66*, 1055–1060. [CrossRef] [PubMed]
20. Xu, R.; Ye, Y.; Zhao, W. Saponins. In *Introduction to Natural Products Chemistry*; CRC Press: Boca Raton, FL, USA, 2012; pp. 125–145.
21. Massin, C.; Uthicke, S.; Purcell, S.W.; Rowe, F.W.E.; Samyn, Y. Taxonomy of the heavily exploited Indo-Pacific sandfish complex (Echinodermata: Holothuriidae). *Zool. J. Linn. Soc.* **2009**, *155*, 40–59. [CrossRef]
22. Matsuno, T.; Ishida, T. Distribution and seasonal variation of toxic principles of sea-cucumber (*Holothuria leucospilota*; Brandt). *Cell. Mol. Life Sci.* **1969**, *25*, 1261. [CrossRef]

23. Van Dyck, S.; Gerbaux, P.; Flammang, P. Elucidation of molecular diversity and body distribution of saponins in the sea cucumber *Holothuria forskali* (Echinodermata) by mass spectrometry. *Comp. Biochem. Physiol. B Biochem. Mol. Biol.* **2009**, *152*, 124–134.
24. Oleszek, W.; Marston, A. *Saponins in Food, Feedstuffs and Medicinal Plants*; Kluwer Academic Publishers: Dordrecht, The Netherlands, 2000; Volume 45.
25. Kalinin, V.I.; Stonik, V.A. Application of morphological trends of evolution to phylogenetic interpretation of chemotaxonomic data. *J. Theor. Biol.* **1996**, *180*, 1–10. [CrossRef] [PubMed]
26. Liu, J.; Yang, X.; He, J.; Xia, M.; Xu, L.; Yang, S. Structure analysis of triterpene saponins in *Polygala tenuifolia* by electrospray ionization ion trap multiple-stage mass spectrometry. *J. Mass Spectrom.* **2007**, *42*, 861–873. [CrossRef] [PubMed]
27. Song, F.; Cui, M.; Liu, Z.; Yu, B.; Liu, S. lMultiple-stage tandem mass spectrometry for differentiation of isomeric saponins. *Rapid Commun. Mass Spectrom.* **2004**, *18*, 2241–2248. [CrossRef] [PubMed]
28. Liu, S.; Cui, M.; Liu, Z.; Song, F.; Mo, W. Structural analysis of saponins from medicinal herbs using electrospray ionization tandem mass spectrometry. *J. Am. Soc. Mass Spectrom.* **2004**, *15*, 133–141. [CrossRef] [PubMed]
29. Zhang, S.Y.; Yi, Y.H.; Tang, H.F.; Li, L.; Sun, P.; Wu, J. Two new bioactive triterpene glycosides from the sea cucumber *Pseudocolochirus violaceus*. *J. Asian Nat. Prod. Res.* **2006**, *8*, 1–8. [CrossRef]
30. Yayli, N.; Findlay, J.A. A triterpenoid saponin from *Cucumaria frondosa*. *Phytochemistry* **1999**, *50*, 135–138. [CrossRef] [PubMed]
31. Wu, J.; Yi, Y.H.; Tang, H.F.; Wu, H.M.; Zou, Z.R.; Lin, H.W. Nobilisides A–C, three new triterpene glycosides from the sea cucumber *Holothuria nobilis*. *Planta Med.* **2006**, *72*, 932–935. [CrossRef] [PubMed]
32. Zhang, S.Y.; Yi, Y.H.; Tang, H.F. Bioactive triterpene glycosides from the sea cucumber *Holothuria fuscocinerea*. *J. Nat. Prod.* **2006**, *69*, 1492–1495. [CrossRef] [PubMed]
33. Liu, B.S.; Yi, Y.H.; Li, L.; Sun, P.; Han, H.; Sun, G.Q.; Wang, X.H.; Wang, Z.L. Argusides D and E, two new cytotoxic triterpene glycosides from the sea cucumber *Bohadschia argus* Jaeger. *Chem. Biodivers.* **2008**, *5*, 1425–1433. [CrossRef] [PubMed]
34. Zhang, S.L.; Li, L.; Yi, Y.H.; Zou, Z.R.; Sun, P. Philinopgenin A, B, and C, three new triterpenoid aglycones from the sea cucumber *Pentacta quadrangularis*. *Mar. Drugs* **2004**, *2*, 185–191. [CrossRef]
35. Kelecom, A.; Daloze, D.; Tursch, B. Chemical studies of marine invertebrates—XX: The structures of the genuine aglycones of thelothurins A and B, defensive saponins of the Indo-pacific sea cucumber *Thelonota ananas* Jaeger (Echinodermata). *Tetrahedron* **1976**, *32*, 2313–2319. [CrossRef]
36. Kitagawa, I.; Kobayashi, M.; Hori, M.; Kyogoku, Y. Marine natural products. XVIII. Four lanostane-type triterpene oligoglycosides, bivittosides A, B, C and D, from the Okinawan sea cucumber *Bohadschia bivittata* mitsukuri. *Chem. Pharm. Bull.* **1989**, *37*, 61–67. [CrossRef]
37. Elyakov, G.B.; Kuznetsova, T.A.; Stonik, V.A.; Levin, V.S.; Albores, R. Glycosides of marine invertebrates. IV. A comparative study of the glycosides from Cuban sublittoral holothurians. *Comp. Biochem. Physiol. B* **1975**, *52*, 413–417.
38. Rothberg, I.; Tursch, B.M.; Djerassi, C. Terpenoids. LXVIII. 23-Acetoxy-17-deoxy-7,8-dihydroholothurinogenin, a new triterpenoid sapogenin from a sea cucumber. *J. Org. Chem.* **1973**, *38*, 209–214. [CrossRef]
39. Girard, M.; Bélanger, J.; ApSimon, J.W.; Garneau, F.X.; Harvey, C.; Brisson, J.R. Frondoside A. A novel triterpene glycoside from the holothurian *Cucumaria frondosa*. *Can. J. Chem.* **1990**, *68*, 11–18. [CrossRef]
40. Yayli, N. Minor saponins from the sea cucumber *Cucumaria frondosa*. *Indian J. Chem. Sect. B* **2001**, *40*, 399–404.
41. Kitagawa, I.; Kobayashi, M.; Son, B.W.; Suzuki, S.; Kyogoku, Y. Marine natural products. XIX: Pervicosides A, B, and C, lanostane-type triterpene-oligoglycoside sulfates from the sea cucumber *Holothuria pervicax*. *Chem. Pharm. Bull.* **1989**, *37*, 1230–1234. [CrossRef]
42. Drozdova, O.; Avilov, S.; Kalinovskii, A.; Stonik, V.; Mil'grom, Y.M.; Rashkes, Y.V. New glycosides from the holothurian *Cucumaria japonica*. *Chem. Nat. Compd.* **1993**, *29*, 200–205. [CrossRef]
43. Wu, J.; Yi, Y.H.; Tang, H.F.; Wu, H.M.; Zhou, Z.R. Hillasides A and B, two new cytotoxic triterpene glycosides from the sea cucumber *Holothuria hilla* Lesson. *J. Asian Nat. Prod. Res.* **2007**, *9*, 609–615. [CrossRef] [PubMed]

44. Rodriguez, J.; Castro, R.; Riguera, R. Holothurinosides: New antitumour non sulphated triterpenoid glycosides from the sea cucumber *Holothuria forskalii*. *Tetrahedron* **1991**, *47*, 4753–4762. [CrossRef]
45. Mimaki, Y.; Yokosuka, A.; Kuroda, M.; Sashida, Y. Cytotoxic activities and structure-cytotoxic relationships of steroidal saponins. *Biol. Pharm. Bull.* **2001**, *24*, 1286–1289. [CrossRef] [PubMed]

marine drugs

Article

A Great Barrier Reef *Sinularia* sp. Yields Two New Cytotoxic Diterpenes

Anthony D. Wright †, Jonathan L. Nielson ‡, Dianne M. Tapiolas, Catherine H. Liptrot § and Cherie A. Motti *

Australian Institute of Marine Science, PMB no. 3, Townsville MC, Townsville, QLD 4810, Australia; adwright@hawaii.edu (A.D.W.); jonathon.nielson@acdlabs.com (J.L.N.); d.tapiolas@aims.gov.au (D.M.T.); catherine.liptrot@jcu.edu.au (C.H.L.)

* Author to whom correspondence should be addressed; c.motti@aims.gov.au; Tel.: +61-7-47534143; Fax: +61-7-47725852.

Received: 4 June 2012; in revised form: 25 June 2012; Accepted: 23 July 2012; Published: 31 July 2012

Abstract: The methanol extract of a *Sinularia* sp., collected from Bowden Reef, Queensland, Australia, yielded ten natural products. These included the new nitrogenous diterpene (4*R**,5*R**,9*S**,10*R**,11*Z*)-4-methoxy-9-((dimethylamino)-methyl)-12,15-epoxy-11(13)-en-decahydronaphthalen-16-ol (**1**), and the new lobane, (1*R**,2*R**,4*S**,15*E*)-loba-8,10,13(14),15(16)-tetraen-17,18-diol-17-acetate (**2**). Also isolated were two known cembranes, sarcophytol-B and (1*E*,3*E*,7*E*)-11,12-epoxycembratrien-15-ol, and six known lobanes, loba-8,10,13(15)-triene-16,17,18-triol, 14,18-epoxyloba-8,10,13(15)-trien-17-ol, lobatrientriol, lobatrienolide, 14,17-epoxyloba-8,10,13(15)-trien-18-ol-18-acetate and (17*R*)-loba-8,10,13(15)-trien-17,18-diol. Structures of the new compounds were elucidated through interpretation of spectra obtained after extensive NMR and MS investigations and comparison with literature values. The tumour cell growth inhibition potential of **1** and **2** along with loba-8,10,13(15)-triene-16,17,18-triol, 14,17-epoxyloba-8,10,13(15)-trien-18-ol-18-acetate, lobatrienolide, (1*E*,3*E*,7*E*)-11,12-epoxycembratrien-15-ol and sarcophytol-B were assessed against three human tumour cell lines (SF-268, MCF-7 and H460). The lobanes and cembranes tested demonstrated 50% growth inhibition in the range 6.8–18.5 μM, with no selectivity, whilst **1** was less active (GI_{50} 70–175 μM).

Keywords: *Sinularia*; Alcyoniidae; anticancer activity; lobane; cembrane; diterpene

1. Introduction

There have been many reports documenting the diversity of secondary metabolites produced by soft corals from the genus *Sinularia*, including sesquiterpenes [1,2], diterpenes [3–7], cembranoids [8–11], polyhydroxylated steroids [12], glycosides [13], sphingosines [14], farnesyl quinols [15,16], and polyamines [17]. These metabolites have been shown to possess a range of biological activities including antimicrobial [5], antiviral [4], anti-inflammatory [4,11], cytotoxic [8–10,17], anticancer [3,18], antifouling [19], antifeedant [20], and allelopathic [21,22] activities. Given this wide-ranging diversity in chemical structure and biological activity, it is not surprising that soft corals, which do not have a hard calcareous skeleton, are relatively well defended against predation [20] and are effective competitors for space on coral reefs [21]. As a result, the *Sinularia* genus remains an attractive target for the discovery of novel bioactive metabolites.

As part of the biodiscovery program at the Australian Institute of Marine Science (AIMS), the ethanol (EtOH) extract of a Great Barrier Reef soft coral *Sinularia* sp., was determined to have significant activity in the NCI 60 cell line COMPARE analysis [23]. Based on this, the sample was selected for recollection, large scale extraction and workup. The methanol (MeOH) extract of the recollected soft coral tissue was subjected to bioassay-guided fractionation, using C18 flash vacuum liquid chromatography and preparative C18 HPLC, to yield the new nitrogenous diterpene (4*R**,5*R**,9*S**,10*R**,11*Z*)-4-methoxy-9-((dimethylamino)-methyl)-12,15-epoxy-11(13)-en-decahydronaphthalen-16-ol (**1**), the new lobane, (1*R**,2*R**,4*S**,15*E*)-loba-8,10,13(14),15(16)-tetraen-17,18-diol-17-acetate (**2**), and eight known diterpenes: two cembranes, sarcophytol-B [24] and (1*E*,3*E*,7*E*)-11,12-epoxycembratrien-15-ol [8], and six known lobanes, loba-8,10,13(15)-triene-16,17,18-triol [25], 14,18-epoxyloba-8,10,13(15)-trien-17-ol [26], lobatrientriol [7], lobatrienolide [7], 14,17-epoxyloba-8,10,13(15)-trien-18-ol-18-acetate [26] and (17*R*)-loba-8,10,13(15)-trien-17,18-diol [27]. The structural elucidation and biological activities of **1**, **2** and of the known compounds loba-8,10,13(15)-triene-16,17,18-triol, 14,17-epoxyloba-8,10,13(15)-trien-18-ol-18-acetate, lobatrienolide, (1*E*,3*E*,7*E*)-11,12-epoxycembratrien-15-ol and sarcophytol-B against a panel of human tumour cell lines are also presented.

2. Results and Discussion

The ^{13}C NMR and ESI-FTMS of **1** established its molecular formula to be $C_{24}H_{43}O_3N$, requiring four degrees of unsaturation. The ^{1}H and ^{13}C NMR spectral data of **1** (Table 1) showed the molecule to contain a trisubstituted double-bond (δ_C 142.5, s, C-11; 117.8, d, C-13; δ_H 5.59, d, 5.2, H-13) as the only multiple bond within the molecule and accounted for one of the degrees of unsaturation. This information, in combination with the molecular formula, showed the molecule to be tricyclic.

Table 1. ^{1}H and ^{13}C NMR data (300 MHz and 75 MHz, CD_3OD) for (4*R**,5*R**,9*S**,10*R**,11*Z*)-4-methoxy-9-((dimethylamino)-methyl)-12,15-epoxy-11(13)-en-decahydronaphthalen-16-ol (**1**).

No.	13C δ (m)	1H δ (m, J Hz)	COSY	gHMBC	nOe
1	42.3 (t)	1.84 (1H, m)	H_b-1, H_b-2	C-10, C-5, C-9, C-2, C-3	
		1.24 (1H, m)	H_a-1, H_a-2, H_b-2	C-5, C-19, C-2	
2	28.1 (t)	1.59 (1H, m)	H_a-1, H_a-3	C-4	
		1.45 (1H, m)	H_a-1	C-10, C-1, C-4	
3	36.3 (t)	1.85 (1H, m)	H_a-2, H_b-3	C-5, C-1, C-4, C-20	
		1.60 (1H, m)	H_b-2, H_a-3	C-5, C-1, C-4	
4	76.8 (s)				
5	53.1 (d)	1.49 (1H, m)	H_2-6	C-6, C-19, C-4, C-20	
6	26.7 (t)	1.82 (2H, m)	H-5, H-7	C-10, C-8	
7	43.1 (d)	1.86(1H, m)	H_2-6	C-5, C-8, C-9	
8	25.0 (t)	1.85 (1H, m)	H_b-8, H-9		
		1.52 (1H, m)	H_a-8	C-10, C-7, C-22	
9	45.2 (d)	1.52 (1H, m)	H_a-22, H_b-22	C-10, C-7, C-22	
10	38.0 (s)				
11	142.5 (s)				
12	69.0 (t)	4.16 (2H, brs)	H-13	C-7, C-11, C-13, C-15	
13	117.8(d)	5.59 (1H, d, 5.2)	H-12, H_a-14, H_b-14	C-7, C-12, C-14, C-15	
14	26.3 (t)	2.12 (1H, m)	H-13, H_b-14, H-15		
		2.00 (1H, m)	H-13, H_a-14, H-15		
15	81.9 (d)	3.25 (1H, m)	H_a-14, H_b-14	C-17, C-18	
16	72.7 (s)				
17	25.2 (q)	1.17 (3H, s)		C-15, C-16, C-18	
18	25.6 (q)	1.17 (3H, s)		C-15, C-16, C-17	
19	15.2 (q)	0.89 (3H, s)			H_b-1, H_b-2, H-20, H_2-22
20	18.7 (q)	1.08 (3H, s)		C-5, C-4, C-3	H_b-1, H_b-2, H-19
21	48.1 (q)	3.16 (3H, s)		C-4	H-5
22	60.5 (t)	3.25 (1H, dd, 3.2, 11.0)	H-9, H_b-22	C-10, C-8, C-9	
		2.93 (1H, dd, 11.0, 13.1)	H-9, H_a-22	C-9	
23	45.2 (q)	2.90 (3H, s)		C-22, C-24	
24	45.2 (q)	2.90 (3H, s)		C-22, C-23	

From the ^1H-^1H COSY spectrum of **1** spin systems from H_b-1 (δ_H 1.24, m) to H_2-3 (δ_H 1.85, m; 1.60, m) via $H_{a/b}$-2 (δ_H 1.59, m; 1.45, m) and from H-5 (δ_H 1.49, m) to H_2-22 (δ_H 3.25, dd, 3.2, 11.0; 2.93, dd, 11.0, 13.1) via H_2-6 (δ_H 1.82, m), H-7 (δ_H 1.86 m), H_2-8 (δ_H 1.85, m; 1.52 m) and H-9 (δ_H 1.52, m) could be discerned. This information together with cross-peaks in the HMBC spectrum from H_b-1 and H-5 to C-19 (δ_C 15.2, q), from H-20 (δ_H 1.08, s) to C-3, C-4 and C-5, and from H-7 to the olefinic C-11 (δ_C 142.5, s), showed the presence of a substituted bicyclic ring system.

The ^1H-NMR spectrum of **1** displayed singlet resonances of a methoxy (-OCH_3) at δ_H 3.16 and an *N*,*N*-dimethyl substituted tertiary amine (-$N(CH_3)_2$) at δ_H 2.90. The HMBC correlation from δ_H 3.16 (s) to δ_C 76.8 (s, C-4) located the methoxy at C-4 while correlations from both H-23/24 to and δ_C 60.5 (C-22) located the tertiary amine at C-22.

Further analysis of the ^1H-^1H COSY indicated the presence of a spin system from δ_H 5.59 (d, 5.2, H-13) to δ_H 3.25 (m, H-15) via δ_H 2.12 and 2.00 (m, H_2-14). HMBC correlations from H-13 to C-7 located the C-11 side chain at C-7 of the bicyclic ring system. Based on HMBC correlations from H_3-17/H_3-18 to δ_C 72.7 (C-16), the two methyl groups with resonances at δ_H 1.17 (H-17/18) were connected to a tertiary carbon bearing an OH, forming a propan-2-ol-2-yl moiety [28]. The data so far accounted for three of the four oxygens, the double-bond, two of the rings, and the nitrogen, leaving one oxygen and one ring unassigned. An ether linkage, forming the third ring, was deduced between C-12 and C-15 based on the HMBC correlation from δ_H 4.16 (brs, H-12) to δ_C 81.9 (C-15), and was further supported by a C-O-C stretch at 1080 cm^{-1} in the IR spectrum of **1**. Hence the planar structure of **1**, a diterpene, is best described as (4*R**,5*R**,9*S**,10*R**,11*Z*)-4-methoxy-9-((dimethylamino)-methyl)-12,15-epoxy-11(13)-en-decahydronaphthalen-16-ol (Scheme 1).

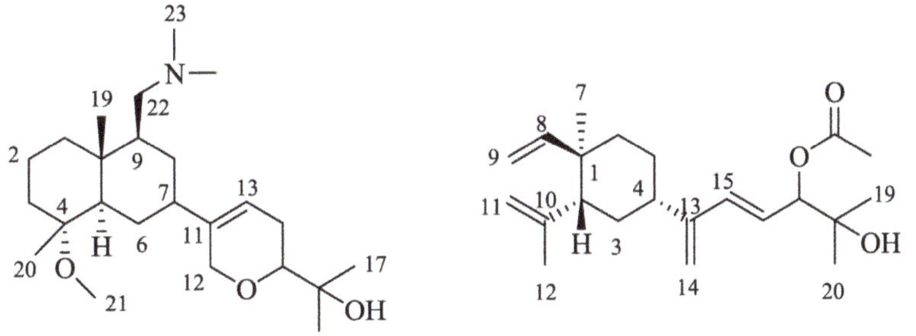

1 **2**

Scheme 1. Structures of (4*R**,5*R**,9*S**,10*R**,11*Z*)-4-methoxy-9-((dimethylamino)-methyl)-12,15-epoxy-11(13)-en -decahydronaphthalen-16-ol (**1**), and (1*R**,2*R**,4*S**,15*E*)-loba-8,10,13(14),15(16)-tetraen-17,18-diol-17-acetate (**2**).

The nOe data of **1** showed correlations between H_3-19 (δ_H 0.89, s) and H_b-1, H_b-2, H_3-20 and H_b-22. These cross peaks revealed the two fused six-membered rings to have a trans-ring junction, CH_3-19 and CH_3-20 to be axial and therefore on the same side of **1**, and the side-chain at C-9 to be on the same side as C-19 (Figure 1). Furthermore, nOe correlations were observed between H_3-21 and H-5 indicating they were on the same side of the molecule as each other but the opposite side of C-19 (Figure 1). The configurations at C-7 and C-15 remain unresolved. Based on the above findings, the relative configurations of chiral carbons C-10, C-5, C-9 and C-4 of **1** were assigned as 4*R**, 5*R**, 9*S** and 10*R** (Scheme 1).

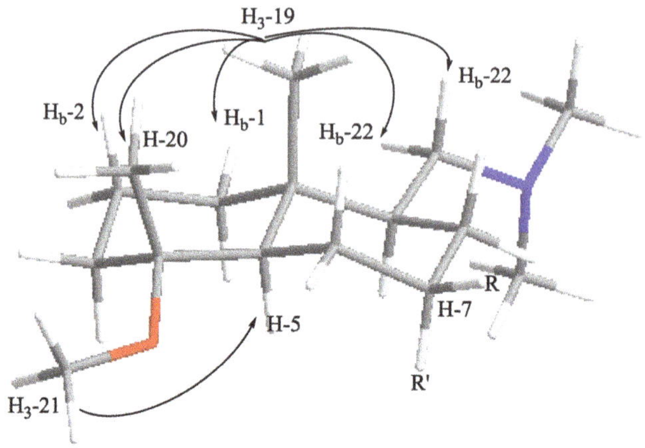

Figure 1. Diagnositic nOe correlations for partial structure of **1**.

The ^{13}C NMR and ESI-FTMS of **2** established its molecular formula as $C_{20}H_{34}O_3$, indicating the molecule to have four degrees of unsaturation. The ^1H and ^{13}C NMR spectral data of **2** (Table 2) showed it contained a vinyl moiety (δ_C 151.6, d, C-8; 110.4, t, C-9; δ_H 5.87, dd, 10.8, 17.6 Hz, H-8; δ_H 4.93, dd, 1.2, 17.6 Hz, H_a-9; δ_H 4.90, dd, 1.2, 10.8 Hz, H_b-9), an isopropenyl group (δ_C 148.9, s, C-10; 112.7, t, C-11, 25.3, q, C-12; δ_H 4.81, brt, 1.5 Hz, H_a-11; 4.59, brs, H_b-11; 1.71, brs, H_3-12) and a tertiary methyl group (δ_C 17.1, q, C-7; δ_H 1.03, s, H_3-7), characteristic of the 3-isopropenyl-4-methyl-4-vinylcyclohexane-1-yl moiety found in lobane-type diterpenoids [7,25–27]. This partial structure was confirmed by analysis of the COSY, HMQC, and HMBC NMR spectral data of **2**. The relative configuration about C-1 and C-2 in **2** was found to be the same as in elemol and several other lobanes, as established by comparison of the ^1H and ^{13}C NMR data for each molecule at centres C-1, C-2, C-6, C-7, C-8, C-9, C-10, C-11 and C-12 [25,27]. Also evident from this data was an exo-methylene (δ_C 151.9, s, C-13; 114.3, t, C-14; δ_H 5.06, s, H_2-14), an endo-disubstituted double-bond (δ_C 137.4, d,C-15; 124.4, d, C-16; δ_H 6.26, d, 16.0, H-15; 5.78, dd, 7.6, 16.0, H-16), a carbonyl group in the form of an acetate (δ_C 172.1, s, O-CO-CH_3; 21.1, q; δ_H 2.09, s, O-CO-CH_3), a CH bearing the acetate (δ_C 82.2, d, C-17; δ_H 5.14, brd, 7.6, H-17), and a propan-2-ol-2-yl moiety the same as that found in **1**. These assignments were corroborated by the IR data with terminal vinyl C-H stretches at 3079 and 3012 cm^{-1}, a carbonyl ester band at 1734 cm^{-1}, and an alcohol OH stretch at 3084 cm^{-1}. This data accounted for all of the remaining unsaturation within the molecule as well as the previously unaccounted for $C_{10}H_{15}O_3$. From the HMBC data of **2** (Table 2), it was evident that C-17 bonded to both C-15 and C-18, as well as the oxygen of the acetyl function. Further, HMBC correlations between H-14 and the carbons C-4, C-13 and C-15, confirmed the side-chain to be attached at C-4 and that the two double-bonds were conjugated, an observation supported by the UV maxima of **2** at 227 nm. With the planar structure of **2** deduced, the double-bond geometry and stereochemistry required resolution. The magnitude of the coupling constant between H-15 and H-16 (J = 16.0 Hz), showed Δ^{15} to have *E* geometry. The relative configurations at C-1 and C-2 were confirmed to be the same as in the known lobane loba-8,10,13(15)-triene-16,17,18-triol [25] on the basis of comparable ^{13}C NMR chemical shift for the same centres. The relative configurations at C-1, C-2 and C-4 were assigned based on NOESY NMR correlations from H-4 to H-2, H_2-5, H_a-6, H-14, H-15, H-16, H_3-19, H_3-20 and O-CO-CH_3, and from H-12 to H-2, H_a-6, H-7, H-8, H_a-9, H_2-11, H_3-19 and confirmed them to be 1*R**, 2*R** and 4*S**, as shown for **2** [6,7,25–27]. The configuration at C-17 remains unresolved. Compound **2** is thus best described as (1*R**,2*R**,4*S**,15*E*)-loba-8,10,13(14),15(16)-tetraen-17,18-diol-17-acetate.

Table 2. ^{1}H and ^{13}C NMR data (300 MHz and 75 MHz, CD_3OD) for (1*R**,2*R**,4*S**,15*E*)-loba-8,10,13(14),15(16)-tetraen-17,18-diol-17-acetate (**2**).

No.	^{13}C δ (m)	^{1}H δ (m, *J* Hz)	COSY	gHMBC	nOe
1	41.0 (s)				
2	54.1(d)	2.13 (1H, m)	H-3	C-1, C-4, C-7, C-10, C-11, C-12	H-4, H-12
3	35.2 (t)	1.66 (2H, m)	H-2, H-4	C-2, C-4	
4	41.5 (d)	2.31 (1H, tdd, 3.4, 4.2, 11.7)	H-3, H$_a$-5, H$_b$-5	C-3, C-13, C-14	H-2, H$_a$-5, H$_b$-5, H$_a$-6, H-14, H-15, H-16, H-19, H-20, O-CO-CH_3
5	28.8 (t)	1.64 (1H, m)	H-4, H$_b$-5, H$_a$-6	C-3	H-4
		1.52 (1H, m)	H-4, H$_a$-5	C-1, C-4	H-2, H-4
6	41.2 (t)	1.60 (1H, m)	H$_a$-5, H$_b$-6	C-1, C-2, C-4, C-5, C-7	H-4, H-12
		1.45 (1H, m)	H$_a$-6	C-2, C-4, C-5	
7	17.1 (q)	1.03 (3H, s)		C-1, C-2, C-6, C-8	H-12
8	151.6 (d)	5.87 (1H, dd, 10.8, 17.6)	H$_a$-9	C-1, C-2, C-6, C-7	H-12
9	110.4 (t)	4.93 (1H, dd, 1.2. 17.6)	H-8, H$_b$-9	C-1, C-2, C-8	H-12, H-17
		4.90 (1H, dd, 1.2, 10.8)	H-8, H$_b$-9	C-1, C-2, C-8	H-17
10	148.9 (s)				
11	112.7 (t)	4.81 (1H, brt, 1.5)	H$_b$-11, H$_3$-12	C-1, C-2, C-10, C-12	H-12
		4.59 (1H, brs)	H$_a$-11, H$_3$-12	C-1, C-2, C-10, C-12	H-12
12	25.3 (q)	1.71 (3H, brs)	H$_a$-11, H$_b$-11	C-1, C-2, C-10, C-11	H-2, H$_a$-6, H-7, H-8, H$_a$-9, H$_a$-11, H$_b$-11, H-19
13	151.9 (s)				
14	114.3 (t)	5.06 (2H, s)		C-4, C-13, C-15, C-16	H-4
15	137.4(d)	6.26 (1H, d, 16.0)	H-16	C-4, C-13, C-14, C-16, C-17	H-4, H-17
16	124.4 (d)	5.78 (1H, dd, 7.6, 16.0)	H-15, H-17	C-13,C-14, C-17, C-18	H-4, H-17
17	82.2 (d)	5.14 (1H, brd, 7.6)	H-16	C-15, C-16, C-18, C-19, C-20, O-CO-CH_3	H$_a$-9, H$_b$-9, H-15, H-16, H-19, H-20, O-CO-CH_3
18	72.7 (s)				
19	25.6 (q)	1.17 (3H, s)		C-17, C-18, C-20	H-4, H-12, H-17, O-CO-CH_3
20	26.2 (q)	1.18 (3H, s)		C-17, C-18, C-19	H-4, H-17, O-CO-CH_3
O-CO-CH_3	172.1 (s)				
O-CO-CH_3	21.1 (q)	2.09 (3H, s)		OAc	H-4, H-7, H-17, H-19, H-20

Complete 1D and 2D NMR data for the known cembranes: sarcophytol-B and (1*E*,3*E*,7*E*)-11,12-epoxycembratrien-15-ol, and the six known lobanes: loba-8,10,13(15)-triene-16,17,18-triol, 14,18-epoxyloba-8,10,13(15)-trien-17-ol, lobatrientriol, lobatrienolide, 14,17-epoxyloba-8,10,13(15)-trien-18-ol-18-acetate and (17*R*)-loba-8,10,13(15)-trien-17,18-diol, are provided for the first time (Supplementary Information). Raju *et al.* reported that loba-8,10,13(15)-triene-16,17,18-triol was the product of long-term, cold storage of the natural product 17,18-epoxyloba-8,10,13(15)-trien-16-ol in $CDCl_3$ [25]. Closer inspection of the FTMS and ^{13}C NMR of the fresh extract in CD_3OD showed the presence of only the triol in our study.

The cytotoxic activities of compounds **1** and **2**, and of the known compounds loba-8,10,13(15)-triene-16,17,18-triol, 14,17-epoxyloba-8,10,13(15)-trien-18-ol-18-acetate, lobatrienolide, (1*E*,3*E*,7*E*)-11,12-epoxycembratrien-15-ol and sarcophytol-B towards a panel of human tumour cell lines are given in Table 3. With the exception of **1** (GI_{50}s all over 70 μM), all compounds showed good activity with GI_{50}s in the range 6.8–18.5 μM. From these data there appears to be no obvious SAR. The four lobanes (including **2**) and the two cembranes all had approximately the same overall activities against the human tumour cell lines SF-268, MCF-7 and H460, with no selectivity.

Table 3. Cytotoxicity data [GI_{50} (μM)] for compounds **1**, **2** and the known compounds loba-8,10,13(15)-triene-16,17,18-triol, 14,17-epoxyloba-8,10,13(15)-trien-18-ol-18-acetate, lobatrienolide, (1*E*,3*E*,7*E*)-11,12-epoxycembratrien-15-ol and sarcophytol-B against the human tumour cell lines SF-268, MCF-7 and H460.

Compound	SF-268 [a]	MCF-7 [b]	H460 [c]
1	175	70	125
2	15	8.8	11.5
Loba-8,10,13(15)-triene-16,17,18-triol	18.5	17	13
Lobatrientriol	NT	NT	NT
14,17-Epoxyloba-8,10,13(15)-trien-18-ol-18-acetate	14	16	18.5
Lobatrienolide	7.4	17	18
14,18-Epoxyloba-8,10,13(15)-trien-17-ol	NT	NT	NT
(17*R*)-Loba-8,10,13(15)-trien-17,18-diol	NT	NT	NT
(1*E*,3*E*,7*E*)-11,12-Epoxycembratrien-15-ol	6.8	12	18.5
Sarcophytol-B	16	12.5	15

[a] SF-268 Central nervous system-glioblastoma cells; [b] MCF-7 Breast-pleural effusion adenocarcinoma cells; [c] H460 Lung-large cell carcinoma cells; NT = Not tested.

3. Experimental Section

3.1. General Experimental Procedures

General experimental procedures are as described previously [29].

3.2. Animal Material

The soft coral *Sinularia* sp., (Order Alcyonacea, Family Alcyoniidae) was collected from the eastern edge of the lagoon at Bowden Reef (19°2.1′S, 147°56.0′E) in the Central Great Barrier Reef, Queensland, Australia, at a depth of 9 m, in June 2005. Collection of this material was conducted under the GBRMPA Permit no. G05/11866.1 and kept frozen (−20 °C) until work-up. A voucher specimen (AIMS 27026) has been lodged with the AIMS Bioresources Library.

3.3. Bioassay

Cellular bioassays were undertaken as described previously [29].

3.4. Extraction and Isolation

Freeze dried animal material (29.6 g) was extracted with MeOH (3 × 400 mL) and a butanol:CH_2Cl_2:H_2O (150:50:100 mL) partition performed. The aqueous phase was further partitioned with BuOH:CH_2Cl_2 (150:50 mL) and the organic phase added to the first organic fraction. The organic fraction (16.8 g) was then subjected to reversed phase C18 flash vacuum chromatography (RP-C18, 25%, 50%, 75%, 100% MeOH in H_2O and 1:1 MeOH:CH_2Cl_2). Activity was observed for the first four fractions. A portion of the 25% MeOH fraction (3.44 g of 10.27 g) was pre-absorbed onto C18, packed into a cartridge, and further separated by preparative C18 HPLC (52 mL/min, isocratic elution at 15% CH_3CN:H_2O for 3 min followed by gradient elution from 15% CH_3CN:H_2O to 100% CH_3CN:H_2O over 50 min and an isocratic elution at 100% CH_3CN for 30 min through a 250 × 41.1 mm Varian Dynamax Microsorb 60-8 C18 column), fractions were collected every 30 s (n = 176) to yield (in order of elution) (4*R**,5*R**,9*S**,10*R**,11*Z*)-4-methoxy-9-((dimethylamino)-methyl)-12,15-epoxy-11(13)-en-decahydronaphthalen-16-ol (**1**, fr 19 and 20 combined, 18.3 mg, 0.06% dry wt of extract), lobatrientriol [7] (fr 71, 24.6 mg, 0.08% dry wt of extract), loba-8,10,13(15)-triene-16,17,18-triol (fr

81, 21.1 mg, 0.07% dry wt of extract), 14,17-epoxyloba-8,10,13(15)-trien-18-ol-18-acetate [26] (fr, 83 and 84 combined, 72.8 mg, 0.07% dry wt of extract), lobatrienolide [7] (fr 87, 24.9 mg, 0.08% dry wt of extract), (1*E*,3*E*,7*E*)-11,12-epoxycembratrien-15-ol [8] (fr 89, 30.9 mg, 0.10% dry wt of extract) and 14,18-epoxyloba-8,10,13(15)-trien-17-ol [26] (fr 109, 123.7 mg, 0.42% dry wt of extract). Fractions 100 to 102 were combined (108.4 mg) and further purified by C18 analytical HPLC (1 mL/min, gradient elution from 5% CH_3CN:H_2O to 100% CH_3CN over 18 min, followed by 6 min with 100% CH_3CN through 250 × 4.6 mm, 5μ Phenomenex Luna (2) C18 column and fractions collected every 30 s) to yield the known compounds (17*R*)-loba-8,10,13(15)-triene-17,18-diol [27] (fr 34, 6.2 mg, 0.02% dry wt of extract) and sarcophytol-B [24] (fr 36, 18.3 mg, 0.06% dry wt of extract) and the new compound (1*R**,2*R**,4*S**,15*E*)-loba-8,10,13(14),15(16)-tetraen-17,18-diol-17-acetate (**2**, fr 33, 2.3 mg, 0.008% dry wt of extract). The known compounds had identical physical and spectroscopic properties to those previously published [7,8,24,26,27].

3.4.1. (4*R**,5*R**,9*S**,10*R**,11*Z*)-4-Methoxy-9-((dimethylamino)-methyl)-12,15-epoxy-11(13)-en-decahydronaphthalen-16-ol (**1**)

Pale yellow oil. $[\alpha]^{24}_D$ +72° (CH_3OH; *c* 0.67); UV (PDA) λ_{max} nm: 195, 208; IR ν_{max} cm^{-1}: 3388, 2969, 2935, 1645, 1468, 1384, 1161, 1080; ^1H (300 MHz, CD_3OD) and ^{13}C (75 MHz, CD_3OD) NMR data Table 1; ESI-FTMS *m/z* $[M + H]^+$ 394.3316 (calcd for $C_{24}H_{44}O_3N$ 394.3303), $[M + Na]^+$ 416.3128 (calcd for $C_{24}H_{43}O_3NNa$ 416.3135).

3.4.2. (1*R**,2*R**,4*S**,15*E*)-Loba-8,10,13(14),15(16)-tetraen-17,18-diol-17-acetate (**2**)

Colourless oil. $[\alpha]^{24}_D$ −9.5° (CH_3OH; *c* 0.23); UV (PDA) λ_{max} nm: 203, 227; IR ν_{max} cm^{-1}: 3408, 2963, 2926, 1734, 1635, 1455, 1372, 1234, 1024, 904; ^1H (300 MHz, CD_3OD) and ^{13}C (75 MHz, CD_3OD) NMR data Table 2; ESI-FTMS *m/z* $[M + Na]^+$ 369.2396 (calcd for $C_{22}H_{34}O_3Na$ 369.2400).

3.4.3. Loba-8,10,13(15)-triene-16,17,18-triol

Colourless oil. ^1H-NMR and ^{13}C-NMR spectral data were consistent with published values [25]; ESI-FTMS *m/z* $[M + Na]^+$ 345.2398 (calcd for $C_{20}H_{34}O_3Na$ 345.2400).

3.4.4. Lobatrientriol

Colourless oil. ^1H-NMR and ^{13}C-NMR spectral data were consistent with published values [7].

3.4.5. 14,17-Epoxyloba-8,10,13(15)-trien-18-ol-18-acetate

Colourless oil. ^1H-NMR and ^{13}C-NMR spectral data were consistent with published values [26].

3.4.6. Lobatrienolide

Colourless oil. ^1H-NMR and ^{13}C-NMR spectral data were consistent with published values [7].

3.4.7. (1*E*,3*E*,7*E*)-11,12-Epoxycembratrien-15-ol

Colourless oil. ^1H-NMR and ^{13}C-NMR spectral data were consistent with published values [8].

3.4.8. 14,18-Epoxyloba-8,10,13(15)-trien-17-ol

Colourless oil. ^1H-NMR and ^{13}C-NMR spectral data were consistent with published values [26].

3.4.9. (17*R*)-Loba-8,10,13(15)-trien-17,18-diol

Colourless oil. ^1H-NMR and ^{13}C-NMR spectral data were consistent with published values [27].

3.4.10. Sarcophytol-B

Colourless oil. ^1H-NMR and ^{13}C-NMR spectral data were consistent with published values [24].

4. Conclusion

Two new compounds, the somewhat unprecedented nitrogen containing (4*R**,5*R**,9*S**,10*R**,11*Z*)-4-methoxy-9-((dimethylamino)-methyl)-12,15-epoxy-11(13)-en-decahydronaphthalen-16-ol (**1**) and the lobane (1*R**,2*R**,4*S**,15*E*)-loba-8,10,13(14),15(16)-tetraen-17,18-diol-17-acetate (**2**), together with the eight known compounds sarcophytol-B [24], (1*E*,3*E*,7*E*)-11,12-epoxycembratrien-15-ol [8], loba-8,10,13(15)-triene-16,17,18-triol [25], 14,18-epoxyloba-8,10,13(15)-trien-17-ol [26], lobatrientriol [7], lobatrienolide [7], 14,17-epoxyloba-8,10,13(15)-trien-18-ol-18-acetate [26] and (17*R*)-loba-8,10,13(15)-trien-17,18-diol [27], were isolated from the Australian soft coral *Sinularia* sp. Although there are many publications detailing the isolation of lobanes [6,7] and cembranes [8,9,11] from soft corals of the genus *Sinularia*, this report shows that new investigations are still yielding further new and somewhat unprecedented derivatives, and that continued investigations of this genus are warranted. The biological and pharmacological properties associated with soft coral chemistry, in particular terpenoids, have been shown to be highly promising [30], leading to the need for more extensive structure-activity relationship studies and further evaluation of their mechanism of action.

Acknowledgments: Collection of this soft coral was made possible through the access and benefit sharing arrangements between AIMS and the Australian Commonwealth Government. The authors are grateful to those AIMS staff, both past and present, involved in the collection. We thank A.-M. Babey, School of Veterinary and Biomedical Sciences, James Cook University for initial cytotoxicity screening data and for the SF-268 cell line and C. Hooi, R. Anderson and C. Cullinane, of the Peter MacCallum Cancer Centre, Melbourne, Australia, for the MCF-7 and H460 cell lines.

References

1. Bowden, B.F.; Coll, J.C.; de Silva, E.D.; de Costa, M.S.L.; Djura, P.J.; Mahendran, M.; Tapiolas, D.M. Studies of Australian soft corals. XXXI. Novel furanosesquiterpenes from several sinularian soft corals (Coelenterata, Octocorallia, Alcyonacea). *Aust. J. Chem.* **1983**, *36*, 371–376. [CrossRef]
2. Park, S.K.; Scheuer, P.J. Isolation and structure determination of two furanosesquiterpenes from the soft coral *Sinularia lochmodes*. *J. Korean Chem. Soc.* **1994**, *38*, 749–752.
3. Radwan, M.M.; Manly, S.P.; Sayed, K.A.E.; Wali, V.B.; Sylvester, P.W.; Awate, B.; Shah, G.; Ross, S.A. Sinulodurins A and B, antiproliferative and anti-invasive diterpenes from the soft coral *Sinularia dura*. *J. Nat. Prod.* **2008**, *71*, 1468–1471.
4. Cheng, S.-Y.; Chuang, C.-T.; Wang, S.-K.; Wen, Z.-H.; Chiou, S.-F.; Hsu, C.-H.; Dai, C.-F.; Duh, C.-Y. Antiviral and anti-inflammatory diterpenoids from the soft coral *Sinularia gyrosa*. *J. Nat. Prod.* **2010**, *73*, 1184–1187. [CrossRef]
5. Aceret, T.L.; Coll, J.C.; Uchio, Y.; Sammarco, P.W. Antimicrobial activity of the diterpenes flexibilide and sinulariolide derived from *Sinularia flexibilis* Quoy and Gaimard 1833 (Coelenterata: Alcyonacea, Octocorallia). *Comp. Biochem. Physiol. Part C* **1998**, *120*, 121–126.
6. Chai, M.-C.; Wang, S.-K.; Dai, C.-F.; Duh, C.-Y. A cytotoxic lobane diterpene from the Formosan soft coral *Sinularia inelegans*. *J. Nat. Prod.* **2000**, *63*, 843–844.
7. Hamada, T.; Kusumi, T.; Ishitsuka, M.O.; Kakisawa, H. Structures and absolute configurations of new lobane diterpenoids from the Okinawan soft coral *Sinularia flexibilis*. *Chem. Lett.* **1992**, *21*, 33–36.
8. Duh, C.-Y.; Hou, R.-S. Cytotoxic cembranoids from the soft corals *Sinularia gibberosa* and *Sarcophyton trocheliophorum*. *J. Nat. Prod.* **1996**, *59*, 595–598. [CrossRef]
9. Duh, C.-Y.; Wang, S.-K.; Tseng, H.-K.; Sheu, J.-H.; Chiang, M.Y. Novel cytotoxic cembranoids from the soft coral *Sinularia flexibilis*. *J. Nat. Prod.* **1998**, *61*, 844–847.
10. Su, J.-H.; Ahmed, A.F.; Sung, P.-J.; Chao, C.-H.; Kuo, Y.-H.; Sheu, J.-H. Manaarenolides A–I, diterpenoids from the soft coral *Sinularia manaarensis*. *J. Nat. Prod.* **2006**, *69*, 1134–1139.
11. Lu, Y.; Huang, C.-Y.; Lin, Y.-F.; Wen, Z.-H.; Su, J.-H.; Kuo, Y.-H.; Chiang, M.Y.; Sheu, J.-H. Anti-inflammatory cembranoids from the soft corals *Sinularia querciformis* and *Sinularia granosa*. *J. Nat. Prod.* **2008**, *71*, 1754–1759.

12. Jagodzinska, B.M.; Trimmer, J.S.; Fenical, W.; Djerassi, C. Sterols in marine invertebrates. 51: Isolation and structure elucidation of C-18 functionalized sterols from the soft coral *Sinularia dissecta*. *J. Org. Chem.* **1985**, *50*, 2988–2992.
13. Kumar, R.; Lakshmi, V. Two new glycosides from the soft coral *Sinularia firma*. *Chem. Pharm. Bull.* **2006**, *54*, 1650–1652. [CrossRef]
14. Subrahmanyam, C.; Kulatheeswaran, R.; Rao, C.V. New sphingosines from two soft corals of the Andaman and Nicobar islands. *Indian J. Chem. Sec. B* **1996**, *35*, 578–580.
15. Cheng, S.-Y.; Huang, K.-J.; Wang, S.-K.; Duh, C.-Y. Capilloquinol: A novel farnesyl quinol from the Dongsha Atoll soft coral *Sinularia capillosa*. *Mar. Drugs* **2011**, *9*, 1469–1476. [CrossRef]
16. Coll, J.C.; Liyanage, N.; Stokie, G.J.; Van Altena, I.; Nemorin, J.N.E.; Sternhell, S.; Kazlauskas, R. Studies of Australian soft corals. III. A novel furanoquinol from *Sinularia lochmodes*. *Aust. J. Chem.* **1978**, *31*, 157–162. [CrossRef]
17. Ojika, M.; Islam, M.K.; Shintani, T.; Zhang, Y.; Okamoto, T.; Sakagami, Y. Three new cytotoxic acylspermidines from the soft coral, *Sinularia* sp. *Biosci. Biotechnol. Biochem.* **2003**, *67*, 1410–1412. [CrossRef]
18. Arepalli, S.K.; Sridhar, V.; Rao, J.V.; Kennady, P.K.; Venkateswarlu, Y. Furano-sesquiterpene from soft coral, *Sinularia kavarittiensis*: induces apoptosis via the mitochondrial-mediated caspase-dependent pathway in THP-1, leukemia cell line. *Apotosis* **2009**, *14*, 729–740. [CrossRef]
19. Mizobuchi, S.; Kon-ya, K.; Adachi, K.; Sakai, M.; Miki, W. Antifouling substances from a Palauan octocoral *Sinularia* sp. *Fish. Sci.* **1994**, *60*, 345–346.
20. Slattery, M.; Hines, G.A.; Starmer, J.; Paul, V.J. Chemical signals in gametogenesis, spawning, and larval settlement and defense of the soft coral Sinularia polydactyla. *Coral Reefs* **1999**, *18*, 75–84. [CrossRef]
21. Sammarco, P.W.; Coll, J.C.; Barre, S.; Willis, B. Competitive strategies of soft corals (Coelenterata: Octocorallia): Allelopathic effects on selected scleractinian corals. *Coral Reefs* **1983**, *1*, 173–178. [CrossRef]
22. Coll, J.C.; Bowden, B.F.; Heaton, A.; Scheuer, P.J.; Li, M.K.W.; Clardy, J.; K., S.G.; Finer-Moore, J. Structures and possible functions of epoxypukalide and pukalide diterpenes associated with eggs of sinularian soft corals (Cnidaria, Anthozoa, Octocorallia, Alcyonacea, Alcyoniidae). *J. Chem. Ecol.* **1989**, *15*, 1177–1191. [CrossRef]
23. Boyd, M.R. The NCI *in-vitro* anticancer drug discovery screen: Concept, implementation and operation, 1985–1995. In *Anticancer Drug Development Guide: Preclinical Screening, Clinical Trials, and Approval*; Teicher, B.A., Ed.; Humana Press: Totowa, NJ, USA, 1997; pp. 23–42.
24. Kobayashi, M.; Nakagawa, T.; Mitsuhashi, H. Marine terpenes and terpenoids I: Structures of four cembrane-type diterpenes; from the soft coral *Sarcophyton glaucum*. *Chem. Pharm. Bull.* **1979**, *27*, 2382–2387. [CrossRef]
25. Raju, B.L.; Subbaraju, G.V.; Rao, C.B.; Trimurtulu, G. Two new oxygenated lobanes from a soft coral of *Lobophytum* species of the Andaman and Nicobar coasts. *J. Nat. Prod.* **1993**, *56*, 961–966.
26. Edrada, R.A.; Proksch, P.; Wray, V.; Witte, L.; van Ofwegen, L. Four new bioactive lobane diterpenes of the soft coral *Lobophytum pauciflorum* from Mindoro, Philippines. *J. Nat. Prod.* **1998**, *61*, 358–361. [CrossRef]
27. Dunlop, R.W.; Wells, R. Isolation of some novel diterpenes from a soft coral of the genus *Lobophytum*. *Aust. J. Chem.* **1979**, *32*, 1345–1351. [CrossRef]
28. Trimurtulu, G.; Faulkner, D.J. Six new diterpene isonitriles from the sponge *Acanthella cavernosa*. *J. Nat. Prod.* **1994**, *57*, 501–506. [CrossRef]
29. Ovenden, S.P.B.; Nielson, J.L.; Liptrot, C.H.; Willis, R.H.; Wright, A.D.; Motti, C.A.; Tapiolas, D.M. Comosusols A–D and comosone A: Cytotoxic compounds from the brown alga *Sporochnus comosus*. *J. Nat. Prod.* **2011**, *74*, 739–743. [CrossRef]
30. Kamel, H.N.; Slattery, M. Terpenoids of *Sinularia*: Chemistry and biomedical applications. *Pharm. Biol.* **2005**, *43*, 253–269.

MDPI
St. Alban-Anlage 66
4052 Basel
Switzerland
Tel. +41 61 683 77 34
Fax +41 61 302 89 18
www.mdpi.com

Marine Drugs Editorial Office
E-mail: marinedrugs@mdpi.com
www.mdpi.com/journal/marinedrugs

www.ingramcontent.com/pod-product-compliance
Lightning Source LLC
LaVergne TN
LVHW070603100526
838202LV00012B/547
* 9 7 8 3 0 3 9 4 3 1 8 8 5 *